MY GURU SAID, "*You don't have to own a thing to enjoy it. It is better to own everything in God.*

"*One evening I was standing alone on a dark street corner in New York, when three hold-up men came up from behind me, one of them pointing a gun.*

" *'Give us your money,' they demanded.*

" *'Here it is,' I said, not at all disturbed. 'But I want you to know that I am not giving it to you out of fear. I have such wealth in my heart that, by comparison, money means nothing to me.' I then gazed at them with God's power, and they were changed.*"

—*from the chapter,* Reminiscences

"*. . . a rich contribution to the spiritual literature of the world*"

"I found *The Path* to be inspirational in the deepest sense, filled with a divine spirit and overflowing to fill the reader with the same blessing. Kriyananda has represented himself and his guru, Paramhansa Yogananda, with joy, with love, and with honor. *The Path* provides clues to the synthesis of East and West, and testifies to the opening of the heart and minds to a new age."

—David Spangler, Author, Lecturer, Findhorn Foundation

"Swami Kriyananda has made a rich contribution to the spiritual literature of the world. *The Path* is an indispensable guidebook in my reference library. I cherish it deeply. I keep a copy in my office and one as a companion on my bedside table at home, and receive great guidance from it."

—Donald Curtis, Minister, Unity Church of Dallas

"A truly great book!"

What Readers Have Said About The Path:

"The Best Ever . . ."

"*The Path* is the most greatly rewarding book I have ever read."

"Electrifying, simply electrifying! There are no biographies to equal this one. I have gone through tomes and tomes. This one ends my search."

"*The Path* is the most beautiful book in my life."

"Couldn't Put It Down . . ."

"My husband and I just buried ourselves in it for three full days. What an inspiration of tears and laughter and joy!"

"I stayed up till 3:30 a.m. reading *The Path*. Swami Kriyananda was telling the story of MY life, and giving me answers where I thought there were only dead ends."

"I can't wait to finish it so I can start it over again!"

"A Joyful Book . . ."

"I never wanted it to end. The writing literally seemed to glow from the pages. I laughed, I wept. Do you realize how astonishingly few books in our entire history of civilization can move one in this manner?"

"I can't help but wonder if in reading your book I am receiving a blessing. Because that is what if feels like."

"I have come upon parts that made me laugh so hard, and parts so tender that I couldn't but cry."

"I Learned So Much . . ."

"The whole world needs this beautiful book. It tells us honestly how one becomes a man of God and that it really happened to a present-day, in-the-flesh human being. It tells, just as in the autobiographies of the Christian saints, of the anxieties, misgivings, triumphs, and the seeming retrogressions, and then the emergence into bright light."

"I think Swami Kriyananda must have lived 'the life of his age.' "

"Open it anywhere and you'll find gems!"

"All the glowing words that could be said wouldn't convey what an enlightening, awakening agent this book is."

"Fascinating, beautifully written, and enormously helpful."

"It should be required reading in schools."

"A Sequel to Yogananda's Autobiography . . ."

"The most inspiring book since *Autobiography of a Yogi*."

"Since *Autobiography of a Yogi*, this is the greatest book I've ever read."

"Swami Kriyananda's book contains the same spirit as Yogananda's autobiography. A fine job."

"I am continually amazed at how Kriyananda conveys through his words such a feeling of Yogananda's presence."

"Yogananda's presence permeates *The Path* as it does his own autobiography."

"A Totally Living Experience . . ."

"I was touched by the openness and honesty, and appreciated so much the wit, humor, and constant streams of helpful insights. More than anything else, I responded to the underlying vibrations of love and joy. Each chapter was an inspiring and uplifting experience."

THE
SHORTENED PATH

Autobiography
of a
Western Yogi

by
Swami Kriyananda

A condensation by the author
of *The Path: Autobiography of a Western Yogi*

Ananda Publications is a supporting industry for Ananda
Cooperative Village, a community of over 200 people founded in
1968 by Swami Kriyananda. We produce and distribute books and
recordings by Swami Kriyananda and members of Ananda on subjects
of personal growth, self-transformation, and simplicity. A free
catalogue is available upon request.

It is our purpose to offer you the inspiration and knowledge you seek
through products of excellence. We promise you prompt and
efficient service, and will answer all personal letters with personal
letters.

Please feel free to write with any questions you may have about our
books, recordings, yoga course, our community or our guest
programs. It is our joy to serve you.

Ananda Publications
14618 Tyler Foote Road
Nevada City, CA 95959

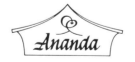

FIRST EDITION © 1977
Shortened Edition © 1981
by Swami Kriyananda

Cover design and photograph by Norman Seeff
All rights reserved
Library of Congress Catalog Card Number: X80-70862
ISBN: 0-916124-19-3
Printed in the United States of America

To the sincere seeker,
whatever his chosen path.

A group of Paramhansa Yogananda's disciples had gone with him to see a movie about the life of Gyandev, a great saint of medieval India. Afterwards they gathered and listened to the Master explain certain, subtler, aspects of that inspiring story. A young man in the group mentioned another film he had seen years earlier, in India, about the life of Mirabai, a famous woman saint.

"If you'd seen *that* movie," he exclaimed, "you wouldn't have even *liked* this one!"

The Guru rebuked him. "Why make such comparisons? The lives of great saints manifest in various ways the same, one God."

OTHER WORKS BY SWAMI KRIYANANDA

Preface

THE TITLE of this shortened edition of *The Path* is intended as a double entendre. It refers not only to the fact that I have condensed that much longer book, but hints also at the truth that one's path to personal fulfillment is much shortened when one seeks *spiritual*, rather than material, achievements.

Part III of this book is completely new, and tells the story of the founding of Ananda Village, in the Sierra Nevada foothills of northern California.

Swami Kriyananda
Ananda Village
California
January 1981

Contents

Part I

Part II

Part III

Illustrations

Part I

Part II

Part III

Introduction

By John W. White, M.A.T., Yale University

author, *Everything You Want to Know About TM*;
editor, *The Highest State of Consciousness*,
Frontiers of Consciousness, *What Is Meditation*;
associate editor, *New Realities Magazine*

WHEN ONE HAS BEEN MOVED to laughter and tears, deep contemplation and joyful insight, as I have been while immersed in *The Path*, it is hardly possible to find a word or a phrase sufficient to encompass the enriching experience.

Briefly, *The Path* is a story of one man's search for God. It serves as a practical manual of instruction for others in search of God-realization, no matter what tradition or path they follow. As an exceptionally lucid explanation of yogic philosophy, *The Path* will also be a valuable resource for those intellectually curious, but not consciously committed to spiritual growth.

Not only is *The Path* inspirational—urging you to "go and do thou likewise"—it also gives the pragmatic technical instruction needed to put principle into action. Moreover, it does so with a beauty and simplicity that is the verbal embodiment of the yogic approach to God-realization. I trust that you will find *The Path* to be a major resource in your life and that you will, in accord with yogic tradition, lovingly share it with others as part of your service to the world. For an inspired work such as this, that is the only proper response.

Cheshire, Connecticut
June 1, 1977

Part I

1

The Pilgrim
Whittles His Staff

THERE ARE TIMES when a human being, though perhaps not remarkable in himself, encounters some extraordinary person or event that infuses his life with great meaning. My own life was blessed with such an encounter nearly thirty years ago, in 1948. Right here in America, of all lands the epitome of bustling efficiency, material progressiveness, and pragmatic "know-how," I met a great, God-known master whose constant vision was of eternity. His name was Paramhansa Yogananda. He was from India, though it would be truer to say that his home was the whole world.

Had anyone suggested to me prior to that meeting that so much radiance, dynamic joy, unaffected humility, and love might be found in a single human being, I would have replied—though perhaps with a sigh of regret—that such perfection is not possible for man. And had anyone suggested to me, further, that divine miracles have occurred in this scientific age, I would have laughed outright. For in those days, proud as I was in my intellectual, Twentieth-Century "wisdom," I mocked even the miracles of the Bible.

No longer. I have seen things that made a mockery of mockery itself. I know now from personal experience that divine wonders do occur on earth. And I believe that the time is approaching when countless men and women will no more think of doubting God than they doubt the air they breathe. For God is not dead. It is man only who dies to all that is wonderful in life when he limits himself to worldly acquisitions and to advancing himself in worldly eyes, but overlooks those spiritual realities which are the foundation of all that he truly *is*.

Paramhansa Yogananda often spoke of America's high spiritual destiny. When first I heard him do so, I marveled. *America?* All that I knew of this country was its materialism, its competitive drive, its smug, "no-nonsense" attitude toward anything too subtle to be measured with scientific instruments. But in time that great teacher made me aware of another aspect, an undercurrent of divine yearning—not in our intellectuals, perhaps, our so-called cultural "leaders," but in the hearts of the common people. Americans' love of freedom, after all, began in the quest, centuries ago, for *religious* freedom. Their historic emphasis on equality and on voluntary, friendly cooperation with one another reflects principles that are taught in the Bible. Americans' pioneering spirit is rooted in these principles.

It was to the divine aspirations of these pioneers of the spirit that Paramhansa Yogananda was responding in coming to America. Americans, he said, were ready to learn the ancient science of yoga.* It was in the capacity of one of modern India's greatest exponents of yoga that he was sent by his great teachers to the West.

In my own life and heritage, the pioneering spirit of America has played an important role. My father, Ray P. Walters, worked for

---

*Yoga: a Sanskrit word meaning, "union." The yogi, a practitioner of the yoga science, acquires both inwardly and outwardly a vision of the underlying unity of all life.

Esso as an oil geologist in foreign lands. Mother, Gertrude G. Walters, after graduating from college, went to study the violin in Paris. My parents were born in Oklahoma; it was in Paris, however, that they met. After their wedding, Dad was assigned to the oil fields of Rumania; there they settled in Teleajen, a small Anglo-American colony about three kilometers east of the city of Ploesti. Teleajen was the scene of my own squalling entrance onto the stage of life.

I came into this world, I believe, already fully myself. I chose this particular family because I found it harmonious to my own nature, and felt that these were the parents who would best afford me the opportunities I needed for my own spiritual development.

Everyone in this world is a pilgrim. He comes alone, treads his chosen path for a time, then leaves once more solitarily. His is a sacred destination, always dimly suspected, though usually not consciously known. Whether deliberately or by blind instinct, directly or indirectly, what all men are truly seeking is Joy—Joy infinite, Joy eternal, Joy divine.

Most of us, alas, wander about in this world like pilgrims without a map. We imagine Joy's shrine to be wherever money is worshipped, or power, or fame, or good times. It is only after ceaseless roaming that, disappointed at last, we pause in silent self-appraisal. And then it is we discover, perhaps with a shock, that our goal was never distant from us at all—indeed, *never any farther away than our own selves!*

The principal purpose of this book is to help you, the reader, to make that discovery. I hope in these pages, among other things, to help you avoid a few of the mistakes I myself have made in the search. For a person's failures may sometimes be as instructive as his successes.

I was born in Teleajen on May 19, 1926, at approximately seven in the morning. James Donald Walters is the full name I received at christening in the little Anglican church in Ploesti. Owing to a plethora of Jameses in the community, I was always known by my second name, Donald, in which I was the namesake of a step-uncle, Donald Quarles, who later served as Secretary of the Air Force under President Eisenhower. James, too, was a family name, being the name of my maternal grandfather. It was my ultimate destiny, however, to renounce such family identities altogether in favor of a higher, spiritual one.

Mother has told me that throughout her pregnancy she was filled with an inward joy. "Lord," she prayed repeatedly, "this first child I give to Thee."

Her blessing may not have borne fruit as early as she had hoped. But bear fruit it did, gradually—one might almost say, relentlessly—over the years.

For mine is the story of one who did his best to live without God, but who—thank God—failed in the attempt.

2

He Sets Out From Home

JOY HAS ALWAYS BEEN my first love. I have longed to share it with others.

My clearest early memories all relate to a special kind of happiness, one that seemed to have little to do with the things around me, that at best only reflected them. For intuitively I felt that there must be some higher reality—another world, perhaps, radiant, beautiful, and harmonious, in relation to which this one represented mere exile.

Often, at night, I would see myself absorbed in a radiant inner light, and my consciousness would seem to expand beyond the limits of my body. "You were eager for knowledge," Mother tells me, "not a little wilful, but keenly sympathetic to the misfortunes of others."

As I grew older, my inner joy spilled over into an intense

enthusiasm for life. More and more, however, I discovered that people often considered my vision of things somewhat peculiar. I was, I suppose, a nonconformist, not from conscious desire or intent, but from a certain inability to attune myself to others' norms. Miss Barbara Henson (now Mrs. Elsdale), our governess for a time, described me in a recent letter the way she remembers me as a child of seven: "You were certainly 'different,' Don—'in the family but not of it.' I was always conscious that you had a mystic quality which set you apart, and others were aware of it, too."

My parents loved us children deeply. Their love for one another, too, was exemplary, and a strong source of emotional security for us. Never in my life have I known them to quarrel, or to have even the slightest falling out. My father was especially wonderful with children. He taught us much, by example as well as words. Above all what we learned from him came from observing in him a nature always humble, honest, truthful, honorable, kind, and scrupulously fair. I would go so far as to call him, in his quiet, rather shy way, a great man.

But in my own relationship with him there was always a certain sadness. I could not be to him the kind of mirror a man naturally hopes for in his sons, especially in his first-born. I tried earnestly to share his interests, but where he was attracted to the "hows" of things, I was attracted to the "whys." He was a scientist, and I, instinctively, a philosopher.

Mother and I understood one another intuitively; ours was a communication of souls, less so of speech. Though she never spoke of praying for us children, I know that her prayers and love for me were my greatest blessing during the formative years of my life.

Rumania was still a feudal land. Its people, gifted artistically, tended otherwise to be somewhat inefficient and unhurried. The country was an anachronism in this busy Twentieth Century. One summer, eager to follow the example of the rest of the modern world, the whole nation went on Daylight *Losing* Time, by official mistake!

Inattention, however, to the petty details of modern commerce and efficiency seemed somehow appropriate in a land that inspired thoughts of music and poetry. Rumania was one of the most fascinatingly beautiful countries I have ever seen: a land of fertile plains and soaring mountains, of colorfully clad peasants and musically gifted gypsies, of hay carts on the highways vying with automobiles for the right of way, of giggling, naked children, of gay songs and laughter. Frequently, outside our colony in the evenings, we would hear bands of gypsies conversing, singing, or playing the violin: the sad, haunting melodies of a people forever outcast from their true home, in India. These gypsies were my first contact with the subtly subjective moods of the Orient—moods that, I was to learn, are reflected in many aspects of life in Rumania. For centuries Rumania had been under Turkish rule. Now a proud and upcoming Western nation, there still clung to her something of the aura of the mystical East.

The church served as a focus for Mother's piety. In this area of her life Dad played the role of disinterested spectator. Though he respected Mother's religious inclinations, and went with her to church more or less regularly, I never observed that liturgy held any attraction for him. His own natural concept of reality was more abstract. Nothing, I think, so inspired him as the contemplation of vast eons of geologic time. The thought of a God sitting somewhere on a heavenly throne, bestowing favors on special groups of worshippers, struck him, I suspect, as faintly barbaric.

My own natural bent lay somewhere between these two, the pious and the abstract. Like Dad, I found it difficult to believe in a God who loved each human being personally. That God was impersonal seemed to me self-evident, when I considered the vastness of the universe. How then, I thought, could He be interested enough to listen to us mortals when we prayed? It was only many years later, in the teachings of India, that I found reconciliation for these seemingly incompatible concepts of a God both personal and impersonal. For the Infinite Spirit, as my guru was to explain with perfect simplicity, though impersonal in its vastness, has become personal also, in creating individual beings. Infinity, in other words, implies infinitesimal littleness as well as infinite immensity.

Every three or four years Dad received a three-months' vacation, all expenses paid, in America. My first journey here was when I was six months old, then three years, seven, ten, and thirteen. It was after I turned thirteen that we settled here.

Vacations in America entailed visits to our various relatives. It was in these relatives, and in many other people like them, that I caught my first glimpse of the particular spiritual genius of America: childlike innocence and simplicity, a predisposition to see goodness in others, a love of freedom tempered by a desire to live in harmony with man and God.

3

Storm Clouds

IT WAS SUMMER, 1935. I was nine years old. Vacationing in the quaint mountain village of Bușteni, I was enjoying a happy season of games, picnics on grassy meadows, and carefree laughter.

One afternoon I went to my room to read a book. Sitting in a chair, I suddenly felt dizzy. I lay down on the bed, but even from this position the room seemed to be spinning. I cried weakly for help, but no one came. At last, summoning all my strength, I struggled to the door, leaning against the wall for support, and called again. This time I was heard.

A doctor was hastily summoned. A large, loud-voiced, over-confident lady, she was evidently determined to prove that I had appendicitis. (*Prod.* "Does it hurt here?" *Prod again.* "How about here?") Minutes of this diagnostic predetermination made me hurt all over. Finally, deciding, perhaps, that it would be no use operating on my entire abdomen, she gave up.

I came near dying in that little village. As it was, though I survived, the happy world I had known for the first nine years of my life died for me with this illness. Back home in Teleajen, all I remember "clearly" are long stretches of delirium.

At last I came to associate *any* unusual mental state with delirium. The very soul-expansion which, until this time, had visited me so often at night, now filled me with a nameless dread.

Because of this fear, I now began making a conscious effort to adjust to the norms of others. For the better part of a decade, insecurity and self-doubt left me anxious to prove to myself that I was not in some indefinable way abnormal.

When I'd recovered sufficiently, my parents decided to send me to a school in the salubrious climate of Switzerland. The school was named, perhaps a trifle pretentiously, *L'Avenir* ("The Future").

My own future here, eighteen long months of it, was somewhat bleak. Only nine years old when I arrived, never before away from my family, and unfamiliar with French (the language commonly spoken at L'Avenir), I was homesick much of the time. Throughout my stay, moreover, I was afflicted with a series of fairly serious illnesses, stemming from my illness which proved to be colitis.

L'Avenir was owned and run by a kindly couple, Mr. and Mrs. John Hampshire. Mr. Hampshire was English; his wife, whom we children knew affectionately as Tante Bea (Aunt Beatrice), was French-Swiss. The students themselves were a mixed bag of Swiss, English, American (me), Italian, and French.

Unhappy though I was, my stay there did have its compensations. The scenery, for one thing, was stunningly beautiful. Across the valley from us loomed the famous Alp, Les Dents du Midi. In winter we skied daily. In warmer weather, frequent walks led us through flowered pastures and quiet, discreet woods—all very properly Swiss.

My long illness coincided with the growing political malady of Europe. In Vienna, where Mother and I stopped on our way to Switzerland, we were warned by friends not to criticize Nazi Germany except in safe places, and then only in whispers. Storm clouds were gathering. In the bluster of bullies everywhere one saw the arrogance of men newly justified in their own eyes. And, growing in the hearts of peace-loving people everywhere, there was fear.

In the summer of 1936 we traveled through Germany on our way to America. A stranger sharing my brother Bob's train compartment was arrested at the German border by the Gestapo. Perhaps he was Jewish. Or perhaps, like thousands of others, he was merely trying to flee despotism. But, young as we were at the time, we knew the likely outcome of his arrest: imprisonment, and then death.

The plight of Europe affected me deeply. Why, I wondered, can't people learn to live together in harmony? What is it in human nature that courts, that seems almost to *demand*, tragedy?

Perhaps my gloomy reflections were aggravated by my own unhappiness. One day I was standing alone on the balcony of our chalet school. Mr. Hampshire came out to find me weeping silently.

"What's the matter?" he inquired gently.

"I'm homesick!" I sobbed.

Kindly, he wrote that day to my parents. Soon it was decided that I should return home.

During my stay in Switzerland Dad had been transferred to Bucharest. Our new residence was on the outskirts of the city at Strada Capitan Dimitriade No. 10. Here I got six months' respite before resuming my formal education. My health through this winter of 1936-37 was still precarious. Occasionally the pain was intense, though I remember now, more clearly than the pain, the tears in Mother's eyes as she suffered with me in her love.

Whether I liked it or not, I now was a little less dependent on the home for which I had so recently been feeling homesick. God was weaning me from dependence on earthly security. My illness; my consequent absence, in that condition, in a far land; my growing sense of aloneness: these were, I think, meant only to help me realize that my true home is not here, on earth, but in Him.

Indeed, this is for all men an eternal truth: God is our reality. Ineluctably we are led, quickly or slowly, by one path or another, towards this divine understanding.

In this thought I am reminded of a brother disciple who once asked our guru, "Will I ever leave the spiritual path?"

"How could you?" the master answered. "Everyone in the world is on the spiritual path."

4

A Temporary Haven

PERHAPS the Divine Fisherman was thinking this poor fish had better not be pulled in too forcibly, lest he break the line. At any rate, the process of dragging me out of my little pond of earthly security became, for a time, relatively pleasant for me. After six months in Bucharest my health was greatly improved. I was eleven years old now, and my parents were anxious to see me resume my formal education.

A Quaker boys' school in England had been highly recommended to us. Nestling snugly in the heart of the Malvern Hills near the village of Colwall, The Downs School was surrounded by verdant, rolling fields, and by narrow country roads that wound their way carefully between clipped, very *English* hedges.

The English have many wonderful traits: honor, loyalty, a sense of duty and fair play. Since, however, this is a chronicle of my spiritual search, I cannot in good conscience ignore what comes across to me as a certain blind spot in their national temperament: a reliance so complete on the ordinary that it gives almost no credence to the extraordinary. Something there is about the religious spirit of England that tries to mold Jesus Christ himself into the very proper image of an English gentleman, and casts the Old Testament prophets as fellow club members with him, perhaps writing occasional letters to the *Times* in protest against the lamentable want of good form in a few of their countrymen. Whether members of the Church of England or of any other sect, the English give one the impression of having neatly clipped and trimmed their religion, like a hedge, to protect values that are primarily social. I refer not to the courageous, free-thinking few, but to the many whose worship seems to close, rather than open, windows onto infinity. I hope I am wrong.

The Downs was easily the best school I ever attended. Religious teaching there may not have been exactly ponderous, but in other respects the teachers knew how to draw the best out of their students. Character building is more basic to the English educational system than to the American. At The Downs, honor, fair play, truthfulness, and a sense of responsibility were given strong emphasis. To tell a lie was considered almost beneath contempt. A boy was once caught stealing sixpence and a little candy from another boy's locker, and so shocked everyone that he was expelled from the school.

In sports, too, though we did our best to win, we were taught that the game itself, not its outcome, was what really mattered. After rugby matches with other schools the members of both teams dined together, rivalry forgotten, new friendships affirmed. I have sometimes wondered what would happen if opposing teams in America were to dine together following a game. Given our national emphasis on winning, I suspect there might be a free-for-all.

The Downs School had a number of innovative features of its own: two kinds of marks, for example, one of them in Greek letters, to show how well we'd done in the subjects themselves; and the other in colors, to show how earnestly we'd applied ourselves to those subjects. Those bright colors seemed somehow even more worth striving for than the letter grades.

Days passed in study, good fellowship, and sports. A fast runner, I managed to play wing three-quarter (the principal running position) in several of the rugby games with other schools. Cricket, however, I considered an utter waste of a sunny afternoon. In practice sessions, which were obligatory, I would lie down in the outfield and wait comfortably for someone to shout, "Walters, get up! The ball's coming your way!"

But while we competed merrily in classrooms and on the playing fields, another more serious conflict was developing in Europe. The relentless approach of World War II made a somber backdrop to our schooldays, one that was never very far from our thoughts. Many of us, we realized, might have to fight in the next war. Many of us would probably be killed.

5

The Storm Breaks

S UMMER CAME, and with it another visit to America. The
weeks passed quietly for us among relatives in Ohio and
Oklahoma. August was about to close its ledger; it was
time for us to return to Europe. We entrained at Tulsa for
New York.

As we stepped out onto the station platform in Chicago, the
headlines struck us with all the force of an ocean wave: *WAR!* Hitler
had invaded Poland. Hopes for peace had been smashed on rocks of
hatred and nationalistic greed. To return now to a war-torn continent
would be foolish. Dad was transferred to the head offices of Esso at
Rockefeller Center in New York City.

We settled eventually in the New York suburb of Scarsdale, at 90
Brite Avenue, in the Foxmeadow section. For the next nine years this

was to be my home, or rather my point of perennial departure.

While I was still a small child my parents had enrolled me at Kent School, in Kent, Connecticut. This was a church school for boys, run by Episcopalian monks. I was not scheduled to enter Kent for another year, however, and was placed meanwhile at Hackley, a boys' school near Tarrytown, New York.

And now the Divine Fisherman began once again to reel in His line determinedly. Looking back after all these years, it is easier for me to summon up a certain proper sense of gratitude to God for holding me so closely in check. At that time, however, I'm afraid gratitude was not my uppermost sentiment. A month earlier my expectations had been glowing. I was returning to The Downs for a happy final year there, surrounded by good friends. Now suddenly I found myself, at thirteen, the youngest boy in the lowest grade of a high school where the only familiar feature was my own perennial status as a "foreigner," a status which, as a born American returning to his own country to live, I found particularly distasteful.

Even my accent, now English, set me apart. But whereas formerly, in England, my American accent had occasioned little more than good-natured amusement, here my English accent marked me for derision. It took me at least a year to learn to "talk American" once again.

Heretofore in my life I had never heard a dirty word. At Hackley it seemed, once I'd been initiated into the new vocabulary, that I heard little else. Aggressive behavior, rudeness, insensitivity to others as an affirmation of one's own independence—these, it seemed, were the norms.

The fact that I was just entering puberty made the problem of adjustment all the more difficult. In truth, I could see no good reason to adjust. Rather, I tended to enclose myself defensively within psychic walls, like a medieval town under attack.

I sought escape in the music room, where for hours at a time I practiced the piano. My unhappiness stirred me also for the first time to a longing for the religious life. Perhaps, I thought, I would become a missionary. I expressed these aspirations, somewhat hesitantly, to my cousin Betty, when both of us were at my parents' home in Scarsdale. She was horrified.

"Not a missionary, Don! There's too much to *do* in this world. You wouldn't want to bury yourself on some primitive island!"

The vigor of her reaction shook me in my still-frail resolution. What, after all, did I really know about the missionary calling? Self-doubt was in any case becoming my own private hell.

After a year at Hackley School, the time came for me to enter Kent.

Kent is an Ivy League prep school that ranks high, scholastically and socially. I entered it with high hopes. But I soon found that the general interests of the boys here were essentially what they had been at Hackley, with the addition of a sort of "All for God, Country, and Our School Team" spirit in which arrogance played the leading part. The Kent student was expected by his peers to embrace every social norm, to like or dislike all the "right" people, and to boast of his proficiency in all the "right" activities. Conformity made one elegible for that supreme reward: popularity. Nonconformity exiled one to a limbo of disapproval and contempt.

I became intensely introverted, miserable with myself. In an environment that demanded absolute conformity, an inability to conform seemed like failure indeed.

I tried my best to enter into the life of the school. I joined the school paper, reporting sports events with a hopeful heart. I joined the debating society. I became a member of the French club. I played football. I rowed. I sang in the glee club.

Nothing worked. There was almost a kind of shame in the few friendships I did form, a tacit understanding that ours was a companionship in failure.

Unhappiness and suffering are necessary for the soul's unfoldment. Without them we might remain satisfied with petty fulfillments. Worse still, we might remain satisfied with *ourselves.**
My personal unhappiness at Kent School inspired me to meditate on the sufferings of mankind everywhere. Could anything, I wondered, be done to improve the human lot?

At fifteen I began writing a novel, about a man who foresaw the destruction of modern civilization, and decided to do what he could to preserve its most constructive elements. Far out into the wilderness he went, and there built a utopian community. The more I thought about my visionary community, the more compellingly it

---

*"Because thou sayest, I am rich, and increased with goods, and have need of nothing; and knowest not that thou art wretched, and miserable, and poor, and blind, and naked: I counsel thee to buy of me gold tried in the fire...and anoint thine eyes with eyesalve, that thou mayest see." (Revelation 3:17,18.)

attracted me. From an escapist dream my concept evolved gradually to a spreading network of intentional villages *within* the framework of present-day civilization. Someday, I resolved, I would start such a community myself.

While I was mentally improving the world, however, my own little world was deteriorating rapidly. A few of the older boys conceived what must have been almost a hatred of me. They began openly threatening to make my life "really miserable" next year, when a few of them would be returning to Kent as student body leaders. In tears that summer I pleaded with Mother to take me home.

I never saw Kent again. Who can say whether I might yet have coaxed a few useful lessons from its dreary walls? But I felt I had taken from them every blessing that I possibly could. I was ready now, inwardly as well as outwardly, for a different kind of schooling.

6

A Paper Rest House: The "Popularity Game"

MOST OF THE YOUNG PEOPLE I met during my adolescence seemed secure in their values. The Nineteen-Forties were unlike the Seventies. Today it is common for young people to question society's values, to seek Meaning, to ponder their relationship to the universe and to God. When I was in high school, as nearly as I could tell I walked alone in such questing.

Others had already planned their lives more or less confidently. They would get good jobs, make money, get ahead in the world, marry, settle down in Scarsdale or in some other wealthy community, raise children, throw cocktail parties, and enjoy the fruits of a normal, worldly life. But I already knew I didn't want money. I didn't want to "get ahead" materially. I wasn't interested in marrying and raising a family. I knew a few of the things I *didn't* want, but had no distinct notion of what it was I *did* want. And in this uncertainty I sometimes doubted whether my disinclination for the things others prized wasn't proof of some inadequacy in myself.

Had others achieved some insight to which I was blind? Certainly my inability to adopt a conventional outlook was a source of intense unhappiness to me.

Now that I had left Kent, and was enrolled as a senior in Scarsdale High School, I determined to overcome what was surely a defect in my character. This new school year, I decided, I would try a great experiment. I would pretend to myself that I *liked* what everyone else liked, that their values were my values, their norms mine. I would see whether, by deliberately adopting their outlook, I could not begin at last to feel at home with it. If I succeeded, how easy my life would become!

As a first step toward "swinging with the crowd," I seized energetically on swing music. Every week I listened eagerly to the radio with my brothers to learn which popular songs had made it onto the Hit Parade. I put on crowd-consciousness like a suit, and soon found that it fit snugly enough. In shouting competitions I pitched in and shouted. In laughing I bubbled with the best. I dated. I danced. I became the vocalist for a local dance band. And as I made a great noise I found, incredibly, that I both liked it and was liked for it.

As months passed it became more and more my second nature to see life in terms of sports, romance, and good times, to laugh with the loudest, roam hither and yon with the most restless, and give and take in the youthful exuberance of an ego competing more or less insensitively with other egos.

Yet somewhere deep inside me a watchful friend remained unimpressed, questioned my motives, observed my follies with detachment, and demanded of me with a sad smile, "Is this what you *really* want?" I was frank enough with myself to admit that it wasn't. Gradually the longing grew within me to stop wasting time.

Questions that had no part in my Great Experiment returned insistently to my mind: What is life? What is the universe? What is the purpose of life on earth? Such issues could not be laughed or shouted away.

7

To Thine Own Search
Be True

I GRADUATED from Scarsdale High School in June, 1943, shortly after turning seventeen. I decided to take advantage of my vacation to broaden my experience of the world.

New York! I worked there as a messenger boy for the *Herald Tribune*. Every day, dodging determined cars, trucks, and buses, and weaving through impatient hordes of shoppers, my fellow messenger boys and I swept pellmell through the rushing bloodstream of big city life. The myriad sense impressions were stimulating, almost overwhelming. In madly bobbing faces on crowded sidewalks, in pleading glances from behind drugstore counters, in fleeting smiles, frosty stares, angry gestures, twitching lips, and self-preoccupied frowns, I saw mankind in virtual caricature, exaggerated out of all credible proportion by the sheer enormity of numbers. Here were tumbling waves of humanity: the youthfully exuberant, the sad and lonely, the stage-struck, the grimly success-oriented, the hard and cynical, the fragile, the lost. All looked hurried and nervous. All seemed harassed by desire.

New York! Its heaving sea of humanity charms and repels in the same instant. It encourages a sense of exaggerated self-importance in those who pride themselves on living in one of the largest, most vital cities in the world. But, in the anonymity it imposes on its faceless millions, it also mocks at self-importance. New Yorkers face a perennial conflict between these opposing challenges to their egos, a conflict that is resolved only by those who seek a broader, spiritual identity. For in the frenzied pace of big-city life it is as if God were whispering to the soul: "Dance with bubbles if you like, but when you tire of dancing, and your bubbles begin bursting one by one, look about you at all these other faces. They are your spiritual brothers and sisters, mirrors to your own self! They *are* you. O little wave, transcend your littleness. Be one with all of them. Be one with life!"

When autumn came I began my higher education at Haverford College, a small men's college on the main line to Paoli from Philadelphia. At that time, owing to the war, it was smaller than ever.

The students were bright-eyed and intelligent; the professors, quiet, sedate, seriously concerned for their students' welfare. Haverford, a Quaker college, conveys the simple, serene dignity that is to be expected of institutions run by that pacific sect. I don't mean we students didn't have our normal boys' share of high times, but these were always inflicted on a background of gentle disapproval from the discreet greystone buildings, and of restrained dismay from our ever-concerned faculty.

We freshmen were so dominant numerically that I actually made the football team. But college sports and I eventually came to a rather cool parting of the ways, due partly to my increasing preoccupation with the search for meaning, and partly, I'm afraid, to the fact that I was attaching "meaning" to a few of the wrong things—like sitting in local bars with friends, nursing a variety of poisonous decoctions, and talking philosophy into the wee hours.

I began devoting much of my free time also to writing poetry, the themes of which related to questions that had long been bothering me: Why suffering? Why warfare and destruction? How is it that God countenances hatred and other forms of human madness? Surely, I thought, suffering can't be His *will* for us? Must it not be a sign, rather, that man is *out of harmony* with God's will?

At this point in my life I might easily have embraced a religious calling. Haverford College is a prominent center of Quakerism. In my time there, leading members of this society were on the faculty: Douglas Steere, Rufus Jones, Howard Comfort. I was impressed by their transparent earnestness and goodness. I also liked the Quaker practice of sitting quietly in meditation at the Sunday services— "meetings," as they were called. Above all, I liked the Quakers for their simplicity. All that they did seemed admirable to me. But somehow I could find no challenge in it. I was seeking a path that would engross me utterly, not one that I could contemplate benignly while puffing on a pipe.

Early during my first semester at Haverford I made friends with Julius Katchen, later famous as a concert pianist. I loved his intensity and enthusiasm. And though I was less agreeably impressed by his egotism, I found compensation for it in his romantic devotion to every form of art, music, and poetry. Our friendship flourished in the soil of kindred artistic interests. In this relationship, Julius was the musician, and I, the poet.

At this time, also, I took a course in poetry composition at nearby Bryn Mawr College under the famous poet, W. H. Auden. Auden encouraged me in my poetic efforts. For some time thereafter, poetry became my god.

Yet there was another side of me that could not remain satisfied for long with Keats's romantic fiction, "Truth is beauty, beauty, truth." In every question, what mattered most to me was not whether an idea was beautiful, but whether in some much deeper sense it was *true*. In this concern I found myself increasingly out of tune with the approach our professors took, which was to view all intellectual commitment with suspicion. Scholarly detachment, not commitment, was their guiding principle.

"That's all very well," I would think. "I want to be objective, too. But I don't want to spend my life sitting on a fence. Even objectivity ought to lead one to conclusions of *some* kind." To my professors, scholarly detachment meant holding a perennial question mark up to life. It meant supporting, "for the sake of discussion," positions to which they didn't really subscribe. It meant showing equal interest in every argument, without endorsing any. I was impatient with their indecisiveness.

It was at about this time that I met a student at Haverford whose search for truth coincided more nearly with my own. Rod Brown was two years older than I, exceedingly intelligent, and a gifted poet. At first our relationship was one of learned sage and unlettered bumpkin of a disciple. Rod treated me with a certain amused condescension, as the ingenuous youngster that I was. My poems he read tolerantly, never lavishing higher praise on them than to call them "nice." *His* poems I couldn't even understand. He would quote at length from countless books I'd never heard of, and could make each quotation sound so important that one got the impression that only a confirmed ignoramus would dare to face life without at least the ability to paraphrase that passage.

Rod was a sensitive young man who had learned early in life to fend off others' rejection of him by treating them with disdain. It was purely a defense mechanism, but he carried it off well. I was as intrigued by his superior attitude towards me for my ignorance as I was captivated by his devotion to philosophical realities. Surely, I thought, if he knew enough to look down on me, it behooved me to learn what the view was from his altitude.

In time we became fast friends. I discovered that, besides his enthusiasm for truth, he had a delightful sense of humor, and was eager to share his ideas and opinions, always fresh and interesting, with others. Rod only raised a supercilious eyebrow at my theories about God, suffering, and eternal life. Rhetorically he would ask, "How can anyone ever know the answers to such questions?" But he directed my thinking constructively into more immediate channels. For the time being the quest for religious truths dropped out of my life. But where the search concerns truth, can *true* religion be very far away?

Rod prompted me to stop concerning myself with life's meaning as an abstraction, and to face the more concrete problem of how to live wisely among men. One of the principles we discussed night after night was nonattachment. Another was the courage to reject values that we considered false, even if all other men believed in them. Amusing as it seems now, we spent hours discussing intellectually the uselessness of intellectualism.

In those days it was Rod who gave me my real education. My classes formed a mere backdrop; they taught me facts, but in discussions with him I learned what I would do with facts. Night after night we sat discussing life over pots of coffee in our rooms, or in bars, or in an off-campus restaurant with the engaging name, "The Last Straw." We had few friends, but that no longer really mattered to me. I was seeking truth now, not the mere opinions of men.

8

Joy Is The Goal

MY FIRST YEAR at Haverford was one of joyous sifting of new ideas. During my second year there, I tried to digest those ideas and make them my own.

I was assigned to a suite in Lloyd Hall, which in normal times was reserved for upper classmen. My roommate was from Argentina. Roberto Pablo Payro was his name. Roberto was quiet, dignified, and ever courteous: ideal qualities in a roommate. He liked sophisticated, serious discussions, mostly on such down-to-earth subjects as politics and sociology, and rather marveled that such abstractions as "life" and "truth" could command from me the intense enthusiasm that they did. My tendency was to seize a thought firmly, wrestle with it for days until I felt I'd mastered it, and then to dash out, laughing, in search of friends with whom I could celebrate my victory. To Roberto I must have seemed alternately far too intense, and inconsistently frivolous.

But thought itself was, for me, a joyous adventure. It was only years later, after I met my guru, that I learned that thinking is but a by-path to truth, and that the highest perceptions are possible only when the fluctuations of the mind have been stilled.

Rod and I had little patience with people who equated seriousness with joylessness. One of our fellow students, with the appropriate last name of Coffin, used to carry a Bible around with him wherever he went, the more sadly to reproach anyone who showed a disposition occasionally to kick up his heels. "The wages of sin," Coffin would remind us gravely, citing chapter and verse, "is death." As my own reputation for cheerful irreverence spread, he took to bringing me the Good News.

If only religion weren't made so lugubrious, I think many people might be inspired to seek God who presently confuse ministers with undertakers. It was years before I myself learned that religious worship needn't verge on the funereal—that it can be, as Paramhansa Yogananda put it, the joyous funeral of all sorrows.

One day at about this time I had what was, to me, a revelation. Sudden, vivid, and intense, it gave me in a few minutes insights into the nature of art and its relationship to truth that have guided my thinking ever since.

The word art, as Rod and I used it, encompassed all the creative arts including music and literature. We had pondered authorities whose claim was that art should be for art's sake alone; or that it must capture reality as a camera does, literally; or that it ought to reflect a sense of social responsibility; or be a purely personal catharsis; or express the spirit of the times in which the artist lives.

Suddenly I felt certain of a truth deeper than all of these. Most artistic theories, I realized, emphasize primarily the forms of art. But art is essentially a human, not an abstract phenomenon. A man's intrinsic worth is determined not by his physical appearance, but by his spirit, his essential attitudes, his courage or cowardice, his wisdom or ignorance. With art, similarly, it is the artist's vision of life, not his medium of expression, that determines the validity of his work. Inspiration, or sterility: Either can be expressed as well through realism as through impressionism. The essential question is: How great does the artist's work reveal HIM to be, as a man? Only if he is great will his work stand a chance of being truly great also. Otherwise it may reveal superlative craftsmanship, but lest plumbers, too, deserve acceptance as artists, mere skill cannot serve to define art.*

My first task as a writer, I decided, was no different from my first task as a human being. It was to determine what constitute ideal human qualities, and then to try to develop *myself* accordingly.

Haverford boys usually dated Bryn Mawr girls. I met a girl at Bryn Mawr named Sue, who came to epitomize for me everything that was good, kind, and holy in life. Her tastes were simple. Her smile expressed so much sweetness that, whether blindly or with actual insight, I could not imagine her holding a mean thought. Our joy in each other's company was such that we never felt the need to go anywhere in particular. A quiet walk through green fields, a friendly chat, a communion of hearts in precious silence: These were the essence of a relationship more beautiful than any I had ever before known.

I had no thought of marriage, of long years spent together, or of anything, really, beyond the present. Sue was for me not so much a girl friend as a symbol of my new gift for giving myself to life joyously, without the slightest thought of return. How she felt toward me seemed almost irrelevant. It was enough, I felt, that my own love for her was true.

Yet there were times, in the happiness of moments together, when she would gaze at me sadly. She wouldn't say why. "Never mind," I would think, "I will only give her the more love, until all her sadness is washed away."

For Christmas I went home. Shortly after the New Year I received a letter from Sue. Eagerly I tore it open.

"Dear Don," it began, "there is something I've been needing to tell you. I realize I should have done so early in our friendship, but I enjoyed your company and didn't want to lose it." She went on to say how deeply she had come to feel about me, and how sad also, that the realities of her life were such that she could never see me again. She was married, she explained, and was even then carrying her husband's baby. Her husband was stationed overseas in the navy. She had realized she would not be allowed to return to college once it

---

*An essay on this subject appears under the title, "Meaning in the Arts," (Ananda Publications, 1978).

became known she was pregnant; hence her resolution of silence. But she had been feeling increasingly unhappy about this resolution insofar as I was concerned. She realized she should have had the courage to tell me sooner. Now she would not be returning to Bryn Mawr to finish the school year. She hoped I would understand the loneliness that had motivated her to go out with me. She had never wanted to hurt me, and was unhappy in the knowledge that such a hurt now was inevitable.

The effect of her letter was devastating. I didn't blame Sue, but rather sympathized with the predicament she'd been in. I reminded myself that I had never asked her to return my love, that in fact I'd never contemplated marriage to anyone. But, oh, the pain!

Much time was to pass before I understood that life, without God, is *never* trustworthy. For God is our only true love. Until we learn to place ourselves unreservedly in His hands, our trust, wherever else we give it, will—*must,* indeed—be betrayed again and again.

9

He Gathers Strength
for the Climb

AT ABOUT THIS TIME in my life I had an interesting dream. I was living with many other people in a torture chamber. For generations our families had lived here, knowing no world but this one; the possibility of any other world simply never occurred to us. One awoke, one was tortured, and at night one found brief respite in sleep. What else could there be to life? We didn't particularly mind our lot. Rather, we imagined ourselves reasonably well-off. Oh, there were bad days to be sure, but then there were also good ones—days together, sometimes, when we were less tortured than usual.

The time came, however, when a handful of us began thinking the unthinkable. Might there, we asked ourselves, just possibly be *another*, a better way of life? Moments snatched when our torturers were out of earshot served to kindle our speculations. At last we determined to rebel.

We laid our plans carefully. One day, rising from our tasks, we slew the torturers and escaped. Slipping out of the great room cautiously, lest armies of torturers be waiting for us outside, we encountered no one. The torture chamber itself, it turned out, occupied only the top floor of a large, otherwise empty building. We walked unchallenged down flights of stairs, emerging from the ground floor onto a vast plain. Confined as we'd been all our lives in the torture chamber, the horizon seemed incredibly distant. Joyfully we inhaled the fresh air. Gazing about us, we all but shouted the new word: Freedom!

Before departing the building forever, we glanced upward to the top floor, scene of the only life we'd ever known. There, to our astonishment, were the very torturers we thought we'd slain, going about their business as though nothing had happened! Amazed, we looked to one another for an explanation.

And then the solution dawned on me. "Don't you see?" I cried. "It's ourselves we've conquered, not the torturers!"

With that realization I awoke.

I felt that this dream held an important meaning for me. The prison, located as it had been on the top floor of the building, symbolized for me the human mind. The torturers represented our mental shortcomings. The emptiness of the rest of the building meant to me that once one overcomes his mental torturers, he finds no more enemies left to conquer. All human suffering, in other words, originates in the mind.

My dream, I felt, held a divine message for me. The time had come for me to seek a higher life. But *how* was I to seek it? I knew nothing of great saints who had communed with God. All I knew of religion were the stylized church services I had attended, the uninspired ministers I had listened to—insecure men who sought support for their faith in the approval of others, not in the unbribable voice of their own conscience.

Though I didn't realize it at the time, my ignorance concerning the spiritual path was my own chief "torturer"; it hindered me from seeking the good for which my soul longed. Subordinate to ignorance there were other, more evident, failings—doubt, for example. Had I approached truth by love I might have gone straight to the mark. But I was trying to *think* my way to wisdom. I had reached a point where I thought about God almost constantly; but He remained silent, for I never called to Him.

I was not yet wise enough to see clearly, but at least my vision was improving. My dream about the torture chamber, conveying as it did a sense of divine guidance, had made me more aware of realities beyond those known through the senses. This awareness led me now to an interesting discovery.

I hit upon what was, as far as I knew then, a novel theory: To be lucky, *expect* luck; don't wait passively for it to come to you, but go out and meet it halfway. With strong, positive expectation, combined with equally positive action, success will be assured. With this simple formula I was to achieve some remarkable results.

Not long after the New Year our first semester ended. At that time Rod, and one or two other friends, flunked out of college. It was hardly surprising, considering the disdain all of us felt for "the system." Their departure put me on my own now in my efforts to understand life more deeply. My independence proved a wholesome opportunity.

My college classes had lost all appeal for me. I seldom mixed with the other students. To protect my unhappiness, I put on an over-intellectual front, did frequent battle with words, and assumed an air of self-assurance in which there was more affirmation than self-recognition. My heart was vulnerable, but not my reason or my will.

Mainly, however, I spent my days thinking, thinking, thinking, as if to wrest from life insights into its farthest secrets. Why was the promise of joy so often a will-o'-the-wisp? And was it not essential to a well-ordered universe that love given be in some way returned? Again, where lay the pathway to true happiness?

"Relax!" cried Roberto one day, seeing me staring sightlessly out the window. "Can't you ever relax!"

So the semester passed, in recollection a grey fog.

As the college year began drawing to a close, my inattention to the daily class routine brought me to a rather awkward predicament. Most of my courses I was at least confident of passing, though barely. Greek, however, was a downright embarrassment. It became a standard joke in class to see whether I would recognize one, or two, Greek words in a paragraph when called upon to translate. The entire semester I did hardly three assignments. As we prepared for the final exam, Dr. Post, our professor, remarked more than once, "Not everyone in this room need trouble himself to appear for that event." Whenever he said this, the other students would glance at me and laugh.

But I determined to show up for the exam, and to pass it. It might take a bit of luck not to flunk, but then, I had my new theory on how to attract luck: *Expect* to be lucky, then meet luck halfway with a vigorous, positive attitude.

Unfortunately, I felt anything but vigorous and positive towards the one activity that really mattered: study. A week before the test I picked up the textbook and glanced half-heartedly at the first page. It was no use. "Tomorrow," I consoled myself, "I'll study *twice* as long as I was going to today." But the next day my good intentions were again routed ignominiously. For the rest of that week I showed persistence only in my continued willingness to procrastinate.

Almost before I knew it, the last evening was upon me. And I hadn't studied at all! Even now I fully intended to pass, but I can't imagine anyone in his right mind endorsing these roseate expectations.

Necessity, it is said, is the mother of invention. Fortunately for me, my present extremity displayed the right, maternal instinct. Out of the blue an inspiration appeared.

"You are a Greek," I told myself with all the concentration I could muster, adjusting myself resolutely to this new identity. The results were astonishing.

As an American, I had found Greek difficult. But now as a Greek "my own" language came surprisingly easily. Through some subtle channel in the network of consciousness that binds all men together, I felt myself suddenly in tune with Greek ways of thinking and speaking. Approaching this new language as an old friend, moreover, I no longer faced the age-old problem of the student who, while attracting knowledge with one half of his mind, pushes it away with the other half by his unwillingness to learn. My entire mental flow was in one direction. For two hours I absorbed Greek grammar and vocabulary like a dry sponge in water, until I could hold no more.

The following morning, "Mother Necessity" gave birth to another inspiration. Our class had been studying the New Testament in the original Greek. Dr. Post had told us that we'd be asked to translate a portion of it into English. This morning, then, mindful of my theory on attracting luck, it occurred to me to turn to the King James translation of the Bible. Only enough time remained for me to read one chapter, but if my luck held, this would be the chapter from which the passage would be selected.

It was! The exam that year as it turned out was exceptionally difficult: Only two students passed it. But my theory on luck was vindicated: I was one of them.

From this experience I learned several useful lessons: for one, the mind's power for positive accomplishment, once it learns to resist its own "no"-saying tendency. Much, indeed, of what people do amounts to pushing simultaneously on opposite sides of a door. Working themselves to exhaustion, they yet accomplish little, or nothing. If they would only learn to say "Yes!" to life with all the conviction of their being, their capacity for success might be expanded almost to infinity.

This discovery was important for me, but even so its interest was secondary to another problem that eluded me still: the secret of happiness.

Is not joy, I asked myself, what all men are really seeking, in their heart of hearts? Why, then, do so few experience it? And why is it so common for people to suffer in the very pursuit of happiness? Toward the end of the semester it occurred to me that perhaps the fault lay with our lifestyle in America. How, I asked myself, could anyone find true happiness while satiating himself on physical comforts? Thoreau's statement in *Walden* impressed me: "Of a life of luxury the fruit is luxury." For the materialist, the heights of inspiration are unimaginable. The worst disease of modern life, I concluded, is complacency. True joy is ever creative; it demands fresh, vital, *intense* awareness. How, I thought impatiently, will happiness worthy of the name ever be felt by people who are too complacent to hold an unconventional thought? Materialism cannot buy happiness.

It is not unusual for this kind of judgment to be met with indulgent smiles, as though the sheer frequency with which it is made, by young people especially, rendered it invalid. But considering the fact that it is arrived at more or less independently by so many seekers after honest values, I think it might be wise to ponder whether it contains an element of truth.

At any rate, my own solution that year to the shortcomings I identified with life in America was to travel abroad. I imagined people in less industrialized countries turning to their daily tasks with a song on their lips, and inspiration in their hearts. Mexico was such a country. I would spend my summer vacation there among simple, happy, spontaneous, *genuine* human beings.

My Mexican adventure proved on the whole exciting, interesting, and fun. I didn't get from it, however, what I'd been seeking most keenly: a better way of life. I'd hoped if nothing else to find more laughter there, more human warmth, more inspiration. For a time I imagined I'd actually found them. But then it dawned on me that what I was experiencing was only my own joyous sense of adventure; the people around me, meanwhile, were engrossed in the same dull round of existence as those back home. Mexicans differed only superficially from Americans; in essence both were the same. They lived, worked, bred, and died; the imaginations of a rare few in either land soared above these mundane activities.

Worse still, from my own point of view, I found that I too was basically no different whether in Villa Obregon and Cuernavaca, or in Scarsdale. I experienced the same physical discomforts, the same need to eat and sleep, the same loneliness. I could appreciate more fully now Thoreau's statement with which he dismissed the common fancy that a person was wiser for having traveled abroad. "I have traveled a good deal," he wrote, "in Concord." He had, too. He knew more about his home town and its environs than any other man alive.

The important thing, I realized, is not what we see around us, but the attitude with which we look. Answers will not be found merely by traveling from one clime to another. To those who expect to find abroad what they have overlooked especially *in themselves*, Emerson's words are a rebuke: "Travel is a fool's paradise."

In college that fall I was discussing with a few friends a movie we'd seen—*The Razor's Edge*, a tale about a Westerner who traveled to India and, with the help of a wise man whom he met there, found enlightenment.

"Oh, if only I could go to India," cried a girl in our group fervently, *"and get lost!"*

I had few illusions left about travel as a solution to the human predicament. "Whom would you lose?" I chuckled. "Certainly not yourself!"

10

Intellectual Traps

A N ANCIENT GREEK MYTH says that Icarus and his father, Daedalus, escaped from Crete on artificial wings fashioned by Daedalus out of wax and feathers. Icarus, over-confident with the joy of flying, ignored his father's advice not to soar too high. As he approached nearer and nearer to the sun, the wax on his wings melted, and Icarus plunged to his death.

Many of the old Greek myths contain deep psychological and spiritual truths. In this one we find symbolized one of man's all-too-frequent mistakes: In his joy at discovering within himself some hitherto unsuspected power, he "flies too high," ignoring the advice of those who have learned from experience to value humility.

I had discovered that, by will power, faith, and sensitive

attunement to certain things that I had wanted to accomplish, I could turn the tide of events to some degree in my favor. But because my enthusiasm was excessive, sensitivity and attunement often got lost in the dust cloud kicked up by my overly affirmative ego.

I wanted wisdom. Very well, then: I *was* wise! I wanted my works to inspire and guide people; I wanted to be a great writer. Very well, then: I *was* a great writer! How simple! All I had to do was some fine day produce the poems, plays, and novels that would demonstrate what was already, as far as I was concerned, a *fait accompli.*

The idea probably had a certain merit, but it was marred by the fact that I was reaching too far beyond my own present realities. In the strain involved there was tension; and in the tension, ego.

Faith, if exerted too far beyond a person's actual capabilities, becomes presumption. Above all it is best always to tie positive affirmations to the whispered guidance of God in the soul. Knowing nothing of such guidance, however, I supplied my own. That which I decreed to be wisdom *was* wisdom. That which I decreed to be greatness *was* greatness. It was not that my opinions were foolish. Many of them were, I believe, fairly sound. But their scope was circumscribed by my own pride. There was no room here for others' opinions. I had not yet learned to listen sensitively to the "truth which comes out of the mouths of babes." Yet I expected ready agreement with my opinions even from those whose age and experience of life gave them some right to consider *me* a babe. I would be no man's disciple. I would blaze my own trails. By vigorous mental affirmation I would bend destiny itself to my will.

Well, I was not the first young man, nor would I be the last, to imagine the popgun in his hand to be a cannon. At least my developing views on life were such that, in time, they refuted my very arrogance.

For my junior year I transferred to Brown University, in Providence, Rhode Island. New perceptions, I felt, would flourish better in a new environment. But my attitude toward formal education was growing increasingly cavalier. I didn't see of what possible use a degree would be to me in my chosen career as a writer.

Most of the writing of my student days has long since been consigned to fire and blessed oblivion. One piece, however, which escaped the holocaust expresses some of my views at that time. It may serve a useful purpose for me to quote it here.

"My countrymen have misunderstood the true meaning of democracy, which is not (as they suppose) to debase the noble man while singing the virtues of the common man, but rather to tell the common man that he, too, can now become noble. The object of democracy is to raise the lowly, and not to praise them for being low. It is only with such a goal that it can have any real merit.

"God's law is right and beautiful. No ugliness exists except man's injustice and the symbols of it. It is not life in the raw we see when we pass through the slums, not the naked truth that many 'realists' would have us see, but the facts and figures of our injustice, the distortion of life and the corruption of truth. If we would claim to be realistic it is not reality we shall see from the squalid depths of humanity, for our view will be premised on injustice and negation. Goodness and beauty will appear bizarre, whereas misery, hatred and all the sad children of man's misunderstanding will seem normal, and yet strange withal and unfounded, as if one could see the separate leaves and branches of a tree and yet could find no trunk. It is not from the hovel of a pauper that we can see all truth, but from the dwelling place of a saint; for from his mountain, ugliness itself is seen, not as darkness, but as lack of light, and the squalor of cities will be no longer foreign, but a native wrong, understood at the core as a symptom of our own injustice.

"The more we watch the outside as a means to understand the inside, the farther off the inside withdraws from our understanding. The same with people as with God."

My ideas were, I think, valid. But ideas alone are not wisdom. Truth must be lived. I'm afraid that, in endless discussions about truth, the sweet taste of it still eluded me.

11

By-Paths

ROD HAD ENROLLED at Boston University. He was as good-humored and intense about everything as ever. Together we devoted much time to a running analysis, complete with droll commentary and merry exaggeration, on some of the follies to which mankind is addicted:

The living-to-impress-others dream: "I work on Wall Street. (*Pause*) Of course, you know what *that* means."

The "Protestant-ethic," I'm-glad-I'm-not-happy-because-that-means-I'm-good dream: "I wouldn't *think* of telling you what you ought to do. All I ask is that you (*sigh*) let your conscience be your guide."

A favorite of ours was the if-you-want-to-be-sure-you're-right-just-follow-the-crowd dream: "You'd better march in step, son, if you want the whole column to move."

Rod was a wonderful mimic. He could make even normally reasonable statements sound ridiculous.

But Rod's life and mine were beginning to branch apart. Rod shared some of my interest in spiritual matters, but not to the extent of wanting to get involved in them himself. I, on the other hand, was growing more and more keen to mold my life along spiritual lines. We talked freely on most subjects, but on this one I found it better to keep my thoughts to myself.

One day I was reading a book, when suddenly I had an inspiration that came, I felt, from some deeper-than-conscious level of my mind. Stunned, I told Rod, "I'm going to be a religious teacher!"

"Don't be silly!" he snorted, not at all impressed.

Very well, I thought, *I'll say no more. But I know.*

The thought of being a religious teacher, however, in no way inspired me to spend more time in church, where religion held no appeal for me whatever. "Hel-*lo!*" our campus minister would simper sweetly, almost embarassingly self-conscious in his effort to demonstrate his "Christian charity" to us when passing us in the hallway. People, I thought, attended church chiefly because it was the respectable and proper thing to do. Some of them, no doubt, wanted to be good, but how many, I wondered, attended because they *loved* God? Divine yearning seemed incompatible, somehow, with going to church, carefully ordered as the services were, and devoid of spontaneity. The ministers in their pulpits talked of politics and sin and social ills—and, endlessly, of money. But they didn't talk of God. They didn't tell us to dedicate our lives to Him. No hint passed their lips that the soul's only true Friend and Lover dwells within, a truth which Jesus stated plainly. Socially inconvenient Biblical teachings, such as Jesus' commandment, "*Leave all,* and follow me," were either omitted altogether from their homilies, or hemmed in with cautious qualifications that left us, in the end, exactly where we were already, armed now with a good excuse.

For years I sought through other channels the fulfillment I craved, because the ministers in their pulpits made a mockery of the very fulfillments promised in the Bible. To paraphrase the words of Jesus, I asked of them the bread of life and they offered me a stone.* An

---

*Matthew 7:9.

emptiness was growing in my heart, and I knew not how to fill it.

My college classes were becoming increasingly burdensome. Intellectualism was not bringing me wisdom. It seemed to me almost unbearably trivial to be studying the Eighteenth-Century novel, when it was the meaning of life itself I was trying to fathom.

Midway through my senior year, I left Brown University.

Thereafter for several months I lived with my parents. I struggled—gamely, perhaps, but without real hope—over a two-act play. It concerned nothing I really wanted to say. But then, the things I did want to way were the last I felt myself decently qualified to express.

Occasionally I went into New York City, and spent hours there walking about, gazing at the tragedy of worldly people's transition from loneliness to apathy. How bereft of joy they seemed, struggling for mere survival in those desolate canyons of concrete!

At other times I would stroll through the happier setting of Washington Square, almost in a kind of ecstasy, observing mothers with babies, laughing children playing on the lawns, young people singing with guitars by the fountain, trees waving, the fountain spray playing colorfully in the sunlight. All seemed joined in a kind of symphony, their many lives but one life, their countless ripples of laughter but one sea of joy.

The valleys and the peaks of life! What grand truth could bind them all together, making them one?

That summer I traveled up to the little town of Putney, Vermont. During my stay there, a drama teacher recommended the Dock Street Theater in Charleston, South Carolina, as a good place to study stagecraft. I decided, albeit in rather a mood of desperation, that if I was going to be a playwright I might as well gain direct experience in the theater.

12

"Who Am I? What Is God?"

I ARRIVED IN CHARLESTON toward the end of June. The Dock Street Theater, I learned, had closed for the summer months, and was not scheduled to open again until September. I took a room in a small boarding house. Most of my fellow boarders were students at The Citadel, a nearby college for men. The friendship of congenial companions my own age threatened for a time my intentions of devoting myself to writing. Rationalizing the threat, I told myself that, as a budding writer, I needed to absorb all I could of local color. I went everywhere, met people in every walk of life, explored various "dives," and was a guest in prominent homes.

Charleston was a small city. I discovered within its narrow boundaries a representative cross section of America. With the middle and upper social strata, and to a lesser degree with the lower, I was already somewhat familiar. But those lower strata which I now encountered were an eye-opener. I'm referring not to the poor, whose simple dignity often gives the lie to that condescending designation, "lower class," but to people, some of them actually wealthy, whose meanness of heart and narrow outlook condemned them to lives of greed.

Many wandered aimlessly from city to city, seeking transient jobs and still more transient pleasures; individuals whose character ,was fast losing distinction in the blur of alcoholic fumes; couples whose family lives were disintegrating under jack-hammer blows of incessant bickering; lonely people who hoped blindly to find in this wilderness of human indifference just a glimpse of friendship.

Everywhere I saw desolation. This, I reflected, was the stuff of which countless plays and novels had been written. Why this preoccupation with negativity? Is great literature something merely to be endured? Who can gain anything worthwhile from exposure to hopelessness?

Yet these, undeniably, were a part of life too. Their effect on me spiritually, moreover, proved to some extent wholesome. For the awareness they gave me of man's potential for self-degradation lent urgency to my own longing to explore a higher potential.

Toward the end of the summer I moved out of my boarding house to a small apartment at 60 Tradd Street. Here I began writing a one-act comedy titled, *Religion in the Park.* Bitter as well as funny, the play concerned a woman who wanted to live a religious life, and who eagerly sought instruction from a priest, only to have him discourage her every devotional sentiment with his careful emphasis on religious propriety. Meanwhile a passing tramp rekindled her fervor with tales of a saint who, he claimed, had cured him of lameness. Here at last was what she'd been seeking: religion *lived,* religion *experienced,* not couched in mere social customs and theoretical dogmas!

But, alas, in the end the tramp proved a fraud. An alcoholic, he had merely invented his tale in the hope of coaxing a few easy dollars into his pocket.

This woman's hope and disillusionment reflected my own longings, and the skepticism that continued to prevent my actual commitment to the religious life.

When the Dock Street Theater opened in September, I went there to seek affiliation with it, but was told that the only way I could do so officially was to enroll as a student in its drama school. Counting myself well out of the academic scene, I asked if I might not be given some other status. Finally the director permitted me, partly on the strength of my new play, to affiliate with them as an "unofficial" student. Under this arrangement I was able to study stagecraft in the evenings, and at the same time to devote my days to writing and thinking.

My probing thoughts, however, led one by one to a dead end. How much, after all, can the theater really accomplish? Did even Shakespeare, great as he was, effect any deep-seated changes in the lives of men? None, surely, at any rate, compared with those which religion has inspired. I shuddered at this comparison, for I loved Shakespeare, and found little to attract me in the churches. But the conclusion, whether I liked it or not, was inescapable: Religion, for all its fashionable mediocrity, remains the most powerfully beneficial influence on earth. Not art, not music, not literature, not science, politics, conquest, or technology: The one truly uplifting power in history, always, has been religion.

How was this possible? Puzzled, I decided to probe beneath the surface, to discover what deep-seated element religion contained that was vital and true.

Avoiding the trap of institutionalized religion, I took to sitting for hours by the ocean, pondering its immensity. I watched little fingers of water rushing in among the rocks and pebbles on the shore. Did God find *personal* expression, similarly, in our own lives?

With ever more pressing urgency the question returned to me: *What IS God?*

One evening, taking a long walk into the gathering night, I deeply pondered this problem. What about thoughtful definitions such as "Cosmic Ground of Being"? No, I thought, the God I was seeking must be a *dynamic force,* one that could transform my life, else there was no point in seeking Him.

Well, then, if He *was* a force, was He a blind force? Surely not, for if God was blind, whence sprang human intelligence?

We all know the signs of exceptional intelligence in man: the bright, alert expression in the eyes, the prompt responses, the general air of competence. An intelligent person may pretend successfully to be stupid, but a stupid person can never successfully pretend to be intelligent. What then of the universe, revealing as it does so many signs of an extraordinary intelligence? The intricate organization of stars, atoms, and creatures, the amazingly exact laws on which the cosmos operates—could a mindless force have created these? Impossible! Rather, human intelligence must be a manifestation, however imperfect, of God!

But then, if to any degree we, in our intelligence, manifest His infinite intelligence, this can only mean that *we are a part of* Him. And then, if life and consciousness are His manifestations, might it not be possible, by deepening our awareness of Him, *to manifest Him more perfectly?* What a staggering concept!

I had spent days watching the ocean surf breaking into long, restless fingers among the rocks and pebbles on the shore. The width of each opening, I now reflected, determined the size of the water's flow. Similarly, if the deepest reality of our lives is God, might it not be possible for us to chip away at the granite of our resistance, and thereby to *widen* our channels of receptivity to Him? And would not His infinite wisdom then, like the ocean, flow into us more abundantly?

If this was true, then, obviously, we should seek above all to develop that aspect of our nature which is closest to God, so that He might enter into and enlighten our consciousness. If we begin there, then perhaps the Divine Ocean will actually assist us to broaden our mental channels.

I realized now that religion is far more than a system of beliefs, and far more than a formalized effort to wheedle a little pity out of God by offering Him pleading, self-condemning prayers and propitiatory rites. If our link with Him lies in the fact that we manifest Him already, *then it is up to us to receive Him ever more perfectly, to express Him ever more fully.** And *this* is what religion is all about! One might, I reflected, devote his entire life to such religion and still have an eternity of development to look forward to. What a thrilling prospect!

This, then, was my calling in life: I would seek God!

Dazed with the grandeur of my reflections, I hardly knew how or at what hour I found my way home again. "Home" at this time was a large, five-room apartment on South Battery which I shared with four of my fellow drama students. On my return there I found them

---

*"But as many as *received* him, to them gave he power to become the sons of God." (John 1:12.)

seated, chatting in the kitchen. More or less automatically, I joined them for a cup of coffee. But my thoughts were far from that convivial gathering. So overwhelmed was I by my new insights that I could hardly speak.

"Look at Don! What's there to be so solemn about?" When they found that I wouldn't participate in their merriment, their laughter assumed a note of mockery.

"Don keeps trying to solve the riddle of the universe! Yuk! Yuk! Yuk!"

"Ah, sweet mystery of life!" crooned another.

"Why, can't you see?" reasoned the fourth, addressing me. "It's all so simple! There's no riddle to be solved! Just get drunk when you like, have fun, shack up with a girl whenever you can, and forget all this craziness!"

"Yeah," reiterated the first, heavily. "Forget it."

To my state of mind just then my roommates sounded like yapping puppies. Of what use to me, such friends? I went quietly to my room.

A few days later I was discussing religion with another acquaintance.

"If you want spiritual teachings," he remarked, "you'll find all your answers in the *Bhagavad Gita.*"

"What's that?" Somehow I found this foreign name strangely appealing.

"It's a Hindu Scripture."

Hindu? I knew nothing of Indian philosophy. But the name, the *Bhagavad Gita,* lingered with me.

If religion was a matter of becoming more receptive to God, it was high time I got busy and did what I could to make myself receptive. But how? It wasn't that I had no idea how to improve myself. Rather, I saw so much room for improvement that I hardly knew where to begin.

Finally I decided that there could be but one way out of my imperfections: God. I must let *Him* guide my life. And what of my plans to be a playwright? Well, what had I been writing, anyway? Could I, who knew nothing, say anything meaningful to others? No, I must give up writing altogether. I must give up my plans to flood the world with my ignorance. Surely, out of very compassion for people I must leave off trying to help them. I must renounce their world, their interests, their attachments, their pursuits. I must seek God in the wilderness, in the mountains, in complete solitude.

I would become a hermit.

I pursued this line of thinking for a time, when a new doubt seized me: Was I losing my mind? Whoever had heard of anyone actually seeking God? I knew nothing as yet about the lives of saints. Vaguely I'd heard them described as people who lived close to God, but the mental image I'd formed of them was of no more than ordinarily good people who went about smiling at children, doing kind deeds, and murmuring, *"Pax vobiscum"* whenever anybody got in their way. What demon of presumption was possessing me that I should be dreaming of actually *finding* God? Surely, I *must* be going mad!

Yet, if this *were* madness, was it not a more solacing condition than the world's vaunted "sanity"? For it was a madness that promised hope, in a world bereft of hope. It was a madness that promised peace, in a world of conflict and warfare. It was a madness that promised happiness, in a world of suffering, cynicism, and broken dreams.

At this point, Reason stepped briskly onto the scene.

"There's nothing wrong with you," it asserted, "that country living can't cure. You've been spending too much time with jaded city people. Get out among simple, genuine, *good* country folk if you want to find peace of mind. Don't waste your life on impossible dreams. Get back to the land! It isn't God you want; it's a more natural way of life, in the harmony and simplicity of Nature."

Ease, in fact, not simplicity, was the heart of this message. For God is so mighty a challenge that the ego will cling to almost anything, rather than heed the call to utter self-surrender.

And, weakling that I was, I relented. I would heed Reason's counsel, I decided. I would go off to the country, commune with Nature, and live among more *natural* human beings.

13

A Search
For Guide-Maps

MY DECISION TO SEEK peace of mind in an environment of bucolic simplicity coincided with the end of the school year, and the closing of the Dock Street Theater for the summer. I returned to New York.

Dad had recently been posted to Cairo, Egypt, as Esso's exploration manager there. Our home in Scarsdale was let, and Mother had taken a house temporarily in White Plains, preparatory to departing for Cairo in August to join Dad. I stayed with her two or three weeks.

My plans for the summer were already set. I said nothing of them, however, to anyone, giving out only that I was going upstate New York; my spiritual longings I kept a carefully guarded secret. But I put in effect immediately my plan to study the Scriptures. Borrowing Mother's copy of the Holy Bible, I began reading it from the beginning.

"In the beginning God created the heaven and the earth. . . . And God said, Let there be light: and there was light." Who is not familiar with these wonderful lines?

"And the LORD God planted a garden eastward in Eden; and there he put the man whom he had formed. . . . And the LORD God commanded the man, saying, 'Of every tree of the garden thou mayest freely eat: But of the tree of the knowledge of good and evil, thou shalt not eat of it: for in the day that thou eatest thereof thou shalt surely die.' "

But—what was this? How could God possibly want man to remain ignorant?

And so man ate the fruit, became wise, and was forced in consequence to live like a witless serf. What kind of teaching was this?

Chapter Five: Here I learned that Adam lived nine hundred and thirty years; his son, Seth, nine hundred and twelve years, and Seth's son, Enos, nine hundred and five years. Cainan, Enos's son, begat Mahalaleel. "And Mahalaleel lived sixty and five years, and begat Jared. . . . And Jared lived an hundred sixty and two years, and he begat Enoch. . . . And Enoch lived sixty and five years, and begat Methuselah. . . . And all the days of Methuselah were nine hundred sixty and nine years: and he died."

What in heaven's name did it all mean? Was some deep symbolism involved?* All this said nothing whatever to my present needs. Disappointed, I put the book down.

In Mother's library there was another book that captured my interest. This one contained brief excerpts from the major religions of the world. Perhaps here I would find the guidance I was seeking.

The selections from the Bible in this book proved more meaningful to me, but even so they seemed too anthropomorphic for my tastes, steeped as I was in the scientific view of reality. The Judaic, the Moslem, the Taoist, the Buddhist, the Zoroastrian—all, I found

---

*Later, when I read my guru's explanation of the story of Adam and Eve, I found its inner meaning profound and deeply inspiring.

poetically beautiful and inspiring, but for me still there was something lacking. I was being asked to believe, but none of these Scriptures, as nearly as I could tell, was asking me to *experience*. Without actual experience of God, what was the good of mere belief? The farther I read, the more all of these Scriptures impressed me as— well, great, no doubt, but at last hopelessly beyond me. Perhaps it was simply a question of style. The standard language of Scripture, I reflected, was cryptic to the point of being incomprehensible.

And then I came upon excerpts from the Hindu teachings—a few pages only, but what a revelation! Here the emphasis was on cosmic realities. God was described as an Infinite Consciousness; man, as a manifestation of that consciousness. Why, this was the very concept I myself had worked out on that long evening walk in Charleston! Man's highest duty, I read, is to attune himself with that divine consciousness: Again, this was what I had worked out! Man's ultimate goal, according to these writings, is to experience that divine reality *as his true Self*. But, how scientific! What infinite promise! Poetic symbolism abounded here, too, as in the other Scriptures, but here I found also explanations, crystal clear and logical. Best of all, I found advice: not only on the religious life generally, but more specifically, on *how to seek God*.

All this was exactly what I'd been seeking! I felt like a poor man who has just been given a priceless gift. Hastily I skimmed through these excerpts; then, realizing the awesome importance they held for me, I put the book aside, and resolved to wait for a later time when I would be free to read these teachings slowly and digest them. Casually I asked Mother if I might take the book upstate with me for the summer. "Of course," she replied, never suspecting the depth of my interest.

My trip upstate New York had been intended, originally, to help me find peace without effort amid the beauties of Nature. But by the time I left White Plains my resolution to work on myself had stiffened markedly. I still hoped that more natural surroundings would contribute something, but I had no illusions that all my answers would be found in a random assortment of hills and trees. God saw to it that *none* of my answers was found there.

As a start toward self-transformation, I decided to begin with vigorous physical discipline. In my initial enthusiasm, of course, I overdid it.

I set out on a one-speed bicycle, taking with me a knapsack that contained only Mother's book of Scriptural excerpts, a few clothes, and a poncho.

My first night I spent in an open field, the poncho spread out underneath me as protection against the damp earth. At three in the morning I awoke, freezing cold, to find myself sloshing about in a puddle of water, collected by my poncho from the heavy dew. Further sleep was impossible. After some time I got up resignedly, and started bicycling again. Mile followed weary mile through deserted mountain terrain, scarcely a village in sight anywhere. Sixteen hours I pedaled that day, mostly uphill, on my one-speed bicycle; I covered well over a hundred miles.

That night I slept twelve full hours.

And so I proceeded, but this time more slowly, to the small mountain town of Indian Lake, where I rented a room and settled eagerly to my reward: a careful study of the excerpts I had from the Indian Scriptures.

14

Joy Is Inside!

Perfect bliss
Grows only in the bosom tranquillised,
The spirit passionless, purged from offense,
Vowed to the Infinite. He who thus vows
His soul to the Supreme Soul, quitting sin,
Passes unhindered to the endless bliss
Of unity with Brahma.

READING THESE WORDS from the *Bhagavad Gita*, my imagination was deeply stirred. The task I faced, as I was learning from the excerpts before me, was to calm my thoughts and feelings, to make myself an open and empty receptacle for God's grace. If I did so, so these teachings stated, God would enter my life and fill it.

All paths, according to the teachings I was reading now, lead by various routes to the same, infinite goal. "As a mother," one stated, "in nursing her sick children, gives rice and curry to one, sago and arrowroot to another, and bread and butter to a third, so the Lord has laid out different paths for different men, suitable to their natures."

How beautiful! How persuasive in its utter fairness!

The Indian teachings stressed the need for testing every Scriptural claim. Direct, personal experience of God, not dogmatic or uncritical belief, was the final test they proposed.

These were the teachings for which I had longed. Too long had I delayed, too long vacillated with doubts, too long sought earthly, not divine, solutions to the deepest problems of life.

One parable in the reading I was engaged in affected me especially. It was from the sayings of a great saint of the Nineteenth Century, Sri Ramakrishna. Not knowing who he was, I imagined the saying was taken from some ancient Scripture.

"How," Sri Ramakrishna asked, "does a man come to have dispassion? A wife once said to her husband, 'Dear, I am very anxious about my brother. For the past one week he has been thinking of becoming an ascetic, and is making preparations for it. He is trying to reduce gradually all his desires and wants.' The husband replied, 'Dear, be not at all anxious about your brother. He will never become a Sannyasin. No one can become a Sannyasin in that way.' 'How does one become a Sannyasin, then?' asked the wife. 'It is done in this way!' the husband exclaimed. So saying, he tore into pieces his flowing dress, took a piece out of it, tied it round his loins, and told his wife that she and all others of her sex were thenceforth mothers to him. He left the house, never more to return."

The courage of this man's renunciation stirred me to the depths.

I now was spending some time every day in meditation. I didn't know how to go about it, but believed that if I could only calm my mind a little bit, I would at least be headed in the right direction.

A local farmer agreed to hire me as a handyman. My intention was to work quietly, thinking of God. But my employer had other, to him infinitely better, ideas: He wanted me to play the fool in his little kingdom. "What else is a handyman for?" he demanded rhetorically, when I remonstrated at being made the constant butt of his rustic jokes. Humor I didn't mind, but I drew the line at *witless* humor. There are few things so exasperating as meeting a gibe with a clever thrust, only to have it soar yards over the other person's head. When, after a few clever sallies, I lapsed resignedly into silence, the farmer teased, "C'mon, flannelmouth! I hired you to *work*. Don't stand there jabbering all day." And that, as I recall, was the high point of his comedy routine. My image of the genuine, innocent, *good* rustic was beginning to fade.

I soon left this worthy's employ. Putting peaceful Indian Lake resolutely behind me, I set off down the road to a succession of similar misadventures.

How, I began to wonder, would I ever become a hermit? A person needed money to buy food. Perhaps, if I could find some place where the money I earned could be stretched farther. . . .

That was it! I would go to some part of the world where the cost of living was low: yes! To South America. I would work in this country first, and save up.

The time finally came for me to return to White Plains and help Mother make preparations for her voyage to Egypt.

My trip south held a certain hope also. A co-worker at a mine had suggested that I might get a job in the merchant marine, where the veriest beginner earned as much as $300 a month. This was good pay in those days. Better still, since I would be out at sea, receiving free board and lodging, I'd be able to save quite a lot of money quickly. I decided to try my luck before the mast.

15

A Map Discovered

O N RETURNING TO White Plains I went to Bowling Green in New York City, and applied for a merchant mariner's card. My hope was to ship out as soon as possible.

Meanwhile I helped Mother pack. When her sailing date came, I accompanied her to the dock in New York and saw her off safely. Next I went down to Bowling Green to see if any ships had come in. No luck: "Come back in a few days." With most of the afternoon still before me, I went uptown to browse at Brentano's, the famous Fifth Avenue book store.

At Brentano's I got into a discussion on spiritual matters with a sales clerk, who showed me a few books by Thomas Merton, the young Protestant Christian who converted to Roman Catholicism,

then went on to become a Trappist monk. I was intrigued, though I
didn't feel personally attracted. It was the catholicity—which is to
say, the *universality*— of India's teachings that had won my devotion.

From Brentano's I went up Fifth Avenue to another book store:
Doubleday-Doran, as it was named then. Here I found an entire
section of books on Indian philosophy—the first I had ever seen.
Hungrily I feasted my gaze on the wide variety of titles: the
Upanishads, the *Bhagavad Gita*, the *Ramayana*, the *Mahabharata*,
books on yoga. I finished scanning these shelves, then turned back to
go over them once again. This time, to my surprise, the first book I
saw, standing face outward on the shelf, was one I hadn't even
noticed the first time. The author's photograph on the cover affected
me strangely. Never had I met anyone whose face radiated so much
goodness, humility, and love. Eagerly I picked up the book and
glanced again at its title: *Autobiography of a Yogi*, by Paramhansa
Yogananda. The author lived in America—in California! Was this
someone at last who could *help* me in my search? As I started to leaf
through the book, these words caught my attention: "Dedicated to the
memory of Luther Burbank, an American saint."

An American *saint?* But, how preposterous! How could anyone
become a saint in this land of the "almighty dollar"? this materialistic
desert? this. . . . I closed the book in dismay, returning it to its place
on the shelf.

That day I bought my first book of Indian philosophy—not
Autobiography of a Yogi, but Sir Edwin Arnold's beautiful translation
of the *Bhagavad Gita*. Eagerly I took this treasure home with me to
Scarsdale, where I had temporarily rented a private room. For the
next couple of days I fairly devoured it, feeling as though I were
soaring in vast skies of pure wisdom.

> By this sign is [the sage] known
> Being of equal grace to comrades, friends,
> Chance-comers, strangers, lovers, enemies,
> Aliens and kinsmen; loving all alike,
> Evil or good.

What wonderful words! Thrilled, I read on:

> Yea, knowing Me the source of all, by Me
>   all creatures wrought,
> The wise in spirit cleave to Me, into My
>   being brought . . .

And unto these—thus serving well, thus
   loving ceaselessly—
I give a mind of perfect mood, whereby they
   draw to Me;
And, all for love of them, within their
   darkened souls I dwell,
And, with bright rays of wisdom's lamp,
   their ignorance dispell.

My own doubts, too, were being dispelled by these marvelous teachings. I knew now with complete certainty that this path was right for me.

The day after I finished my first reading of the *Bhagavad Gita*, I returned to New York, intending to visit Bowling Green and see if any ship had come in. I was walking down Seventh Avenue toward the subway, the entrance to which was on the far side of the next cross street, when I recalled the book I'd rejected so summarily on my last visit to the city: *Autobiography of a Yogi*. As I remembered that beautiful face on the cover, a strong urge from within prompted me to go buy it. I thrust the thought firmly out of my mind.

"That isn't what I'm looking for," I told myself. Chuckling, I added, "An American saint, indeed!" Resolutely I continued walking toward the subway.

At that moment I reached the corner. I was proceeding toward the curb ahead of me when I felt as though an actual force were turning me left around the corner, and propelling me toward Fifth Avenue. I'd never experienced anything like it before. Amazed, I asked myself, "Is there something in this book that I'm *meant* to read?" Resisting no longer, I hastened eagerly in the direction of Doubleday-Doran's.

Entering the store, I made straight for the book and bought it. As I was turning to leave, I bumped into a friend from Scarsdale High School days. He began describing to me in glowing terms his plans for making a career in radio and advertising. The longer he talked, the more closely I hugged this increasingly precious book to my heart. Imperceptibly, my doubts about it had already vanished. Suddenly this oriental yogi and I were old friends. The world and I were strangers, but here was one who knew me, and understood.

I waited until I reached my room in Scarsdale before opening the book. And then began the most thrilling literary adventure of my life.

Autobiography of a Yogi is the story of a young Indian's intense search for God. It describes, more clearly than any other mystical work I have ever read, the author's own experiences with God, including the highest one possible, *samadhi,* or mystical union. In chapter after chapter I read of intense love for God such as I myself yearned to possess; of a relationship with the Lord more intimate, more dear than I had dared to imagine possible.

Until now I had supposed that a life of devotion might give one, at best, a little peace of mind. But here, suddenly, I discovered that the fruit of spiritual living is a joy beyond human imagination!

Never before had I encountered a spirit so clearly truthful, so filled with goodness and joy. Every page seemed radiant with light. Reading *Autobiography of a Yogi,* I alternated between tears and laughter: tears of pure joy; laughter of even greater joy! For three days I scarcely ate or slept. When I walked it was almost on tiptoe, as though in an ecstatic dream.

What this book described, finally, was the highest of sciences, Kriya Yoga, a technique that enables the seeker to advance rapidly on the path of meditation. I, who wanted so desperately to learn how to meditate, felt all the excitement of one who has found a treasure map, the treasure in this case being a divine one buried deep within my own self!

Autobiography of a Yogi is the greatest book I have ever read. One perusal of it was enough to change my entire life. I resolved in the smallest detail of my life to follow Paramhansa Yogananda's teaching.

The day after finishing the book I packed my bag, entrained for New York, and took the next westward-bound bus available.

My break with the past was sudden and complete.

16

The Pilgrim
Meets His Guide

I ARRIVED IN LOS ANGELES on the morning of Saturday, September 11, 1948, exhausted from my long journey. There I took advantage of the first opportunity I'd had in four days to shave and bathe, then continued by bus one hundred miles south to Encinitas, the little coastal town where, as I had read, Yogananda had his hermitage. In the fervor of first reading it had somehow eluded me that he had founded a world-wide organization. Perhaps I had subconsciously "tuned out" this information from my long-standing fear of religious institutionalism. In my mind, this little seaside hermitage was all that existed of his work.

I arrived in Encinitas late that afternoon, too tired to proceed at once to the hermitage. I booked into a hotel and fairly collapsed onto my bed, sleeping around the clock. The next morning I set out for the

Self-Realization Fellowship hermitage, walking perhaps a mile past picturesque gardens, colorful with ice plant and bougainvillea. Many of the flowers I saw there were new to me. The vividness of their hues made a vigorous contrast to the more conservative flowers in the East—a contrast, I was to discover, that extended to numerous other aspects of life on the two coasts.

I approached the hermitage with bated breath. Yogananda, I recalled from his book, once visited a saint without sending prior notice that he was coming. He hadn't yet reached the saint's village when the man came out to welcome him. Did Yogananda, too, I asked myself, know I was coming? And would he, too, come out and greet me?

No such luck. I entered the grounds through an attractive gate, to find on both sides of the driveway a large, beautifully kept garden— trees to the left, a wide lawn to the right. At the far end of the driveway stood a lovely white stucco building with a red tile roof. I imagined disciples quietly going about inside, doing simple chores, their faces shining with inner peace. (Did *they* know I was coming?)

I rang the front door bell. Minutes later a gentle-looking elderly lady appeared.

"May I help you?" she inquired politely.

"Is Paramhansa Yogananda in?"

My pronunciation of this unfamiliar name must have left something to be desired. The white palm beach suit I was wearing, moreover, didn't mark me as the normal visitor. I'd assumed, mistakenly, that palm beach was the accepted attire in southern California, as it was in Miami or Havana. My unusual appearance, together with my obvious unfamiliarity with Yogananda's name, must have given the impression that I was a serviceman of some sort.

"Oh, you've come to check the water?"

"No!" Gulping, I repeated, "Is Paramhansa Yogananda in?"

"Who? Oh, yes, I see. No, I'm afraid he's away for the weekend. Is there anything I can do for you?"

"Well, yes. No. I mean, I wanted to see *him.*"

"He's lecturing today at the Hollywood church."

"You have a *church* there?" I'd always imagined that Hollywood consisted of nothing but movie studios. My astonishment must have struck my hostess as unseemly. After all, why *shouldn't* they have a church in a big city like Hollywood? Soon it became apparent to me that I wasn't making the best possible impression.

Well, I thought, perhaps it *did* seem a bit strange, my barging in here and asking to speak to the head of the organization, and—worse still—not even realizing that he *had* an organization. My hostess drew herself up a little stiffly.

"I want to join his work," I explained. "I want to live here."

"Have you studied his printed lessons?" she inquired, a bit coolly I thought.

"Lessons?" I echoed blankly. "I didn't know he had any lessons to be studied." My position seemed to be getting murkier by the minute.

"There's a full course of them. I'm afraid you couldn't join," she continued firmly, "until after you'd completed the lot."

"How long does that take?" My heart was sinking.

"About four years."

Four years! Why, this was out of the question! As I look back now on that meeting, I think she was probably only trying to temper what, to her, must have seemed my absurd presumption in assuming I had merely to appear on the scene to be welcomed joyously with cries of, "You've arrived!" In fact, the requirement for joining was not so strict as she made it out to be. But it is usual, and also quite proper, for the spiritual aspirant's sincerity to be tested.

It looked less than proper to me at the time, however. It was only later that I learned that my hostess had been Sister Gyanamata, Paramhansa Yogananda's most advanced woman disciple. She herself, it happened, because she had been married, had had to wait years before she could enter the hermitage. The mere *prospect* of a wait must not have seemed to her very much of a test.

Well, I reflected rebelliously, this wasn't *Yogananda's* verdict. Choking down my disappointment, I inquired how I might get to the Hollywood church. Sister Gyanamata gave me the address, and a telephone number. Soon I was on my way back to Los Angeles.

On the way there I alternated between bouts of heated indignation (at *her* presumption!) and desperate prayers for my acceptance. This was the first time in my life I had wanted anything so desperately. I couldn't, I simply *mustn't* be refused.

At one point, thinking again of my elderly hostess, my mind was about to wax indignant once more when suddenly I remembered her eyes. They had been very calm—even, I reflected with some astonishment, wise. Certainly there was far more to her than I'd realized. "Forgive me," I prayed, "for misjudging her. It was wrong of me in any case to think unkindly of her. She was only doing her duty. But I see now that she is a great soul. Forgive me."

A cloud seemed suddenly to lift inside me. I knew in my heart that I'd been accepted.

Arrived in Los Angeles, I checked my bag at the bus depot, and proceeded at once to 4860 Sunset Boulevard, where the church was located. It was about three o'clock in the afternoon. The morning service had long since ended, and, apart from a small scattering of people, the building was empty. A lady greeted me from behind a long table at the back of the room.

"May I help you?"

I explained my mission.

"Oh, I'm afraid you couldn't possibly see him today. His time is completely filled."

I was growing more desperate by the minute. "When *can* I see him?"

She consulted a small book before her on the table. "His appointments are fully booked for the next two and a half months." *Two and a half months!* First I'd been told I couldn't join for four years. Now I was told I couldn't even *see* him for. . . .

"But I've come all the way from New York just for this!"

"Have you?" She smiled sympathetically. "How did you hear about him?"

"I read his autobiography a few days ago."

"So recently! And you came—just—like that?" She cooled a little. "Usually people write first. Didn't you write?"

Bleakly I confessed I hadn't even thought of doing so.

"Well, I'm sorry, but you can't see him for another two and a half months. In the meantime," she continued, brightening a little, "you can study his lessons, and attend the services here."

Morosely I wandered about the church, studying the furnishings, the architecture, the stained-glass windows. It was an attractive chapel, large enough to seat over one hundred people, and invitingly peaceful. An excellent place, I thought, for quiet meditation. But my own mind was hardly quiet or meditative. It was in turmoil.

"You *must* take me!" I prayed. "You *must!* This means my whole life to me!"

Two or three of the people sitting in the church were monks whose residence was the headquarters of Self-Realization Fellowship on Mt. Washington, in the Highland Park section of Los Angeles. I spoke to one of them. Norman his name was; tall and well-built, his eyes were yet gentle and kind. He talked a little about their way of life at Mt. Washington, and their relation, as disciples, to Paramhansa Yogananda. "We call him, 'Master,' " he told me. From

Autobiography of a Yogi I knew already that this appellation, which Yogananda used also in reference to his own guru, denoted reverence, not menial subservience.

How Norman's description of Mt. Washington attracted me! I simply *had* to become a part of this wonderful way of life. It was where I belonged. It was my home.

Norman pointed out two young men sitting quietly farther back in the church.

"They want to join, too," he remarked.

"How long have they been waiting?"

"Oh, not long. A few months."

Disconsolately I wandered about awhile longer. Finally it occurred to me—novel thought!—that perhaps I simply wasn't ready, and that for this reason the doors weren't opening for me. If this were true, I decided, I'd just go live in the hills near Hollywood, come to the services regularly, study the lessons, and—I sighed—wait. When I was ready, the Master would know it, and would summon me.

With this resolution in mind, and with no small disappointment in my heart, I made for the door.

No doubt I'd needed this lesson in humility. Perhaps things had always gone too easily for me. Perhaps I was too confident. At any rate, the moment I accepted the thought that I actually might not be spiritually ready, the situation changed dramatically. I had reached the door when the secretary—Mary Hammond, I later learned her name was—came up from behind me.

"Since you've come such a long way," she said, "I'll just ask Master if he'd be willing to see you today."

She returned a few minutes later.

"Master will see you next."

Shortly thereafter I was ushered into a small sitting room. The Master was standing there, speaking to a disciple in a white robe. As the young man was about to leave, he knelt to touch the Master's feet. This was, I knew from Yogananda's book, a traditional gesture of reverence among Indians; it is bestowed on parents and other elders as well as on one's guru. A moment later, the Master and I were alone.

What large, lustrous eyes now greeted me! What a compassionate smile! Never before had I seen such divine beauty in a human face. The Master seated himself on a chair, and motioned me to a sofa beside him.

"What may I do for you?" For the third time that day, these same, gentle words. But this time how fraught with meaning!

"I want to be your disciple!" The reply welled up irresistibly from my heart. Never had I expected to utter such words to another human being.

The Master smiled gently. There ensued a long discussion, interspersed by long silences, during which he held his eyes half open, half closed—"reading" me, as I well knew.

Over and over again in my heart I prayed desperately, "You *must* take me! I know that you know my thoughts. I can't say it outwardly; I'd only weep. But you must accept me. You *must!*"

Early in the conversation he told me, "I agreed to see you only because Divine Mother told me to. I want you to know that. It isn't because you've come from so far. Two weeks ago a lady flew here all the way from Sweden after reading my book, but I wouldn't see her. I do only what God tells me to do." He reiterated, "Divine Mother told me to see you."

"Divine Mother," as I already knew from reading his book, was the way he often referred to God, Who, he said, embraces both the male and the female principles.

There followed some discussion of my past. He appeared pleased with my replies, and with my truthfulness. "I knew that already," he once remarked, indicating that he was only testing me to see if I would answer him truthfully. Again a long silence, while I prayed ardently to be accepted.

"I am taking fewer people now," he said.

I gulped. Was this remark intended to prepare me for a letdown?

I told him I simply could see nothing for myself in marriage, or in a worldly life. "I'm sure it's fine for many people," I said, "but I don't want it for myself."

He shook his head. "It isn't as fine for *anybody* as people like to make out. God, for everyone, is the *only* answer!" He went on to tell me a few stories of the disillusionments he had witnessed. Then again, silence.

At one point in our discussion he asked me how I had liked his book.

"Oh, it was wonderful!"

"That's because it has my vibrations in it," he replied simply.

Vibrations? I'd never thought of books as possessing "vibrations" before. But, clearly, I had found his book almost alive in its power to convey, not merely ideas, but new states of awareness.

Incongruously, even absurdly, it now occurred to me that he might be more willing to take me if he felt I could be of some practical use to his work. And what did I know? Only writing. But that, surely, was better than nothing. Perhaps he had a need for people with writing skills. To demonstrate my ability, I said:

"Sir, I found several split infinitives in your book." A twenty-two-year-old, literarily untried, but already a budding editor! I've never lived down this faux pas! But Master took it with a surprised, then a humorous, smile. The motive for my remark was transparent to him.

More silence.

More prayers.

"All right," he said at last. "You have good karma. You may join us."

"Oh, but I can wait!" I blurted out, hoping he wasn't taking me only because I hadn't yet found any other place to stay.

"No," he smiled. "You have good karma, otherwise I wouldn't accept you."

Gazing at me with deep love, he then said, "I give you my unconditional love."

Immortal promise! I couldn't begin to fathom the depth of meaning in those marvelous words.

"Will you give me your unconditional love?"

"Yes!"

"And will you also give me your unconditional obedience?"

Desperate though my desire was to be accepted by him, I wanted to be utterly honest. "Suppose," I asked, "sometime, I think you're wrong?"

"I will never ask anything of you," he replied solemnly, "that God does not tell me to ask." He continued:

"When I met my master, Sri Yukteswar, he said to me, 'Allow me to discipline you.' 'Why, Sir?' I inquired. 'Because,' he answered, 'in the beginning of the spiritual path one's will is guided by whims and fancies. Mine was, too, until I met my guru, Lahiri Mahasaya. It was only when I attuned my will to his wisdom-guided will that I found true freedom.' In the same way, if you will tune your will to mine, you, too, will find freedom. To act only on the inspiration of whims and fancies is not freedom, but bondage. Only by doing God's will can you become truly free."

"I see," I replied thoughtfully. Then from my heart I said, "I give you my unconditional obedience!"

My guru continued: "When I met my master, he gave me his unconditional love as I have given you mine. He then asked me to love him in the same way, unconditionally. But I replied, 'Sir, what if

I should ever find you less than a Christlike master? Could I still love you in the same way?' My master looked at me sternly. 'I don't want your love,' he said. 'It stinks!' "

"I understand, Sir," I assured him. He had struck at the heart of my greatness weakness: intellectual doubt. With deep feeling I said to him, "I give you my unconditional love!"

He went on to give me various instructions.

"Now, then, come kneel before me."

I did so. He made me repeat, in the name of God, Jesus Christ, and our line of gurus, the vows of discipleship and of renunciation. Next he placed the forefinger of his right hand on my chest, over the heart. For at least two minutes his arm vibrated, almost violently. Incredibly, from that moment onward, my consciousness, in some all-penetrating manner, was transformed.

I left his interview room in a daze. Norman, on hearing the news of my acceptance, embraced me lovingly. It was unusual, to say the least, for a disciple to be accepted so soon. A few moments later, Master came out from behind the open curtain on the lecture platform. Smiling at us quietly, he said:

"We have a new brother."

Part II

1

My parents, Ray and Gertrude Walters, in Teleajen, Rumania a few days after my appearance on the scene, May, 1926.

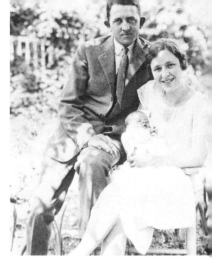

2

A typical scene of rural Rumania as it was when I lived there.

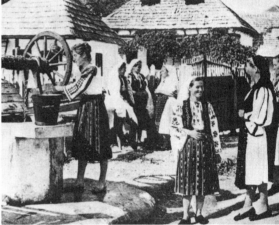

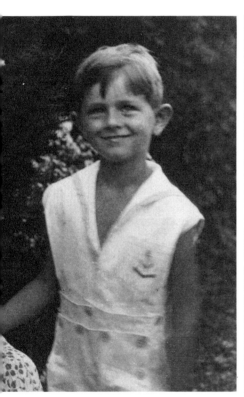

3

Myself at the age of five.

4

In Bucharest, when I was ten.

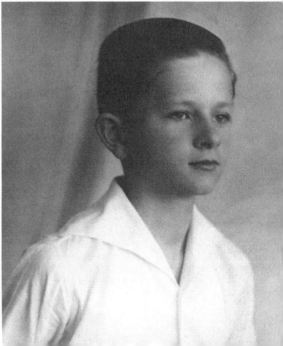

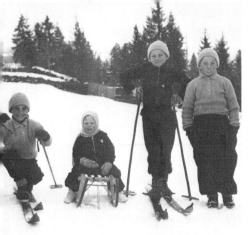

5

With schoolmates at L'Avenir, my Swiss school. I am second from the right.

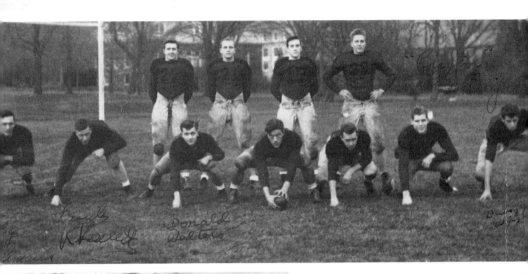

6

Our football team at Haverford, 1943. Because of my size, our college paper referred to me as a "watch charm guard," but we managed to do well.

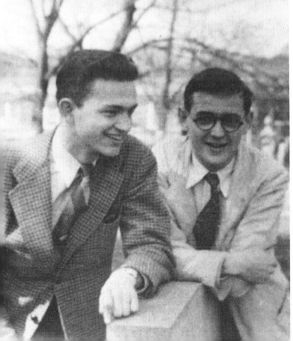

7

My college friend, Rod Brown, and I near his home in Wellesley, Massachusetts.

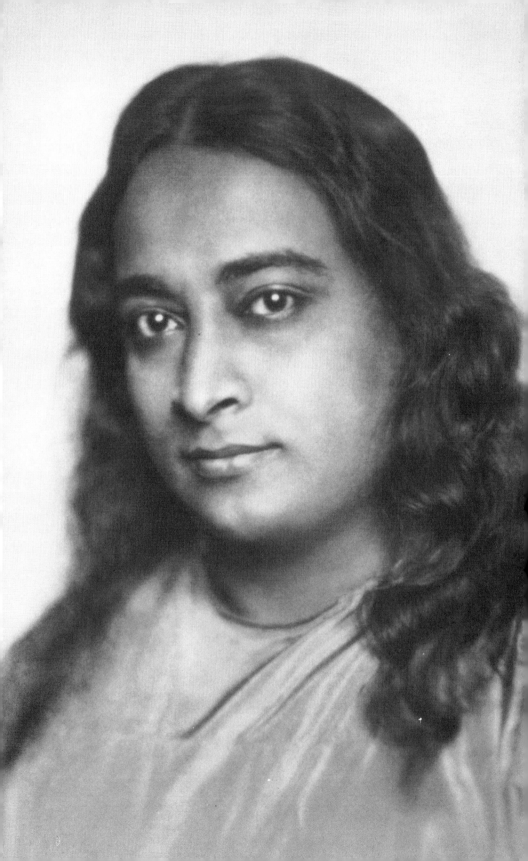

ever had I met anyone whose face radiated so much goodness, humility, and love."

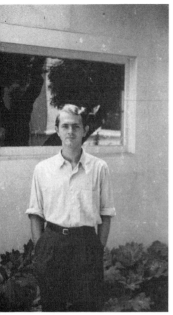

9

In front of my cottage at Mt. Washington, in the autumn of 1949.

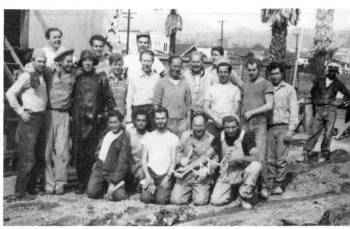

10

The monks working on building India Center, in 1951. *back row:* Second from left, Norman Paulsen; far right, Roy Eugene Davis, who has since become a well-known writer and teacher. *middle row:* Sixth from left, Jean Haupt; third from the right, Joe Carbone (Brother Bimalananda); second from the right, Henry Schaufelberger (Brother Anandamoy). *front row:* Second from left, Debi Mukherjee; next to the right, me.

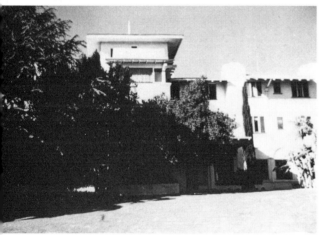

11

Mt. Washington Estates, headquarters of Self-Realization Fellowship. Top floor extreme right, Master's sitting room; to the left of it, his bedroom. Partly framed by the trees at left, his interview room.

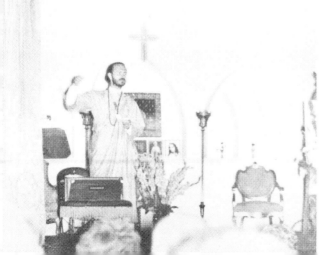

12

I conducted services in the SRF Hollywood church from 1949 to 1958, and was the minister there from 1955 onwards.

13

Christmas at Mt. Washington, 1949. St. Lynn (Rajarsi Janakananda), Master, and Dr. Lewis are seated at the table. Mrs. Lewis is standing behind St. Lynn. I am standing in the background.

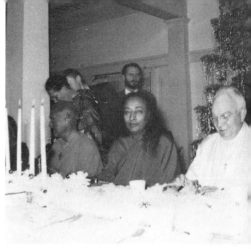

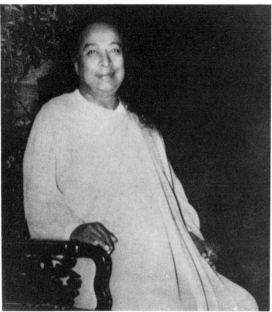

14

Master exemplified the androgynous balance of the perfect human being. He had the compassion and love of a mother, and the wisdom and will power of a father. Here the mother aspect is exemplified.

15

Paramhansa Yogananda in the garden of his Encinitas Hermitage.

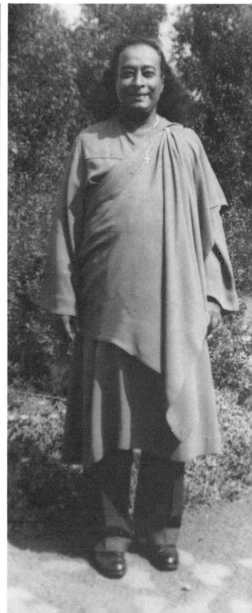

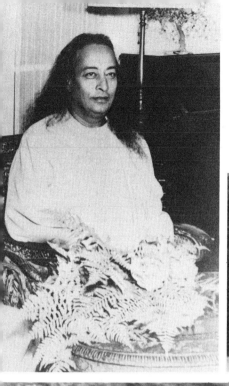

16

"It was clear that Master enjoyed things not for their own sake, but because they manifested in various ways his one, infinite Beloved. Often, as he was expressing joy outwardly, I would note in the still depths of his gaze a fathomless detachment."

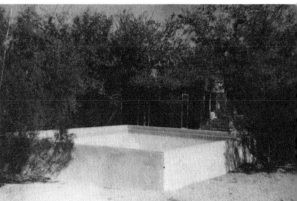

17

Master's retreat at Twenty-Nine Palms.

18

August, 1951. At the time this photograph was taken, Master was suffering from an illness that had affected his legs, and he was unable to walk. He was scheduled to speak to a large convocation of members. Unwilling to publicize his condition, he determined to walk when the time came. A car took him near the outdoor lecture platform. Master lifted his legs with his own hands, and placed both feet on the ground. "Instantly a brilliant light surrounded my body," he later told us. "I was able to walk with ease." We saw him go up onto the platform, stand through his long lecture, and walk back, unaided, to the car. "Once back in the car," he told us, "my legs became helpless again."

19

"I will always love you," said Master to an old detractor.

20

His words had a profound influence. Here flanking Master are Ambassador and Mrs. Binay R. Sen, taken three days before Master's passing. To the right of Ambassador Sen is Mr. M.R. Ahuja, Consul General of India in San Francisco; peering over the two Indians at the right is Dick Haymes, the well-known singer and actor whom I initiated into Kriya Yoga.

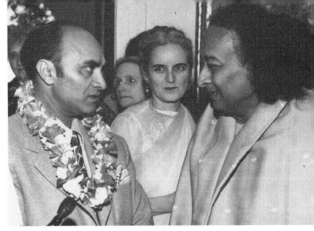

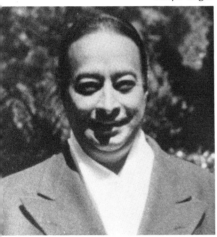

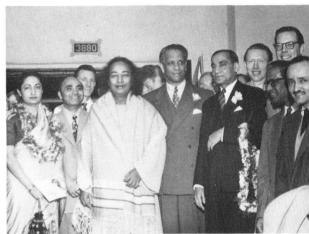

21

Master's everyday attire was a business suit. His desire was not to "Indianize" Americans, but to help them spiritualize their own culture. He tied his long hair back in a bun so that it was hardly noticeable.

22

Master chanting "Om" with his hands raised, registered his thoughts in the ether. After a lecture in Beverly Hills, California, 1950: "We must go on—not only those who are here, but thousands of youths must go North, South, East and West to cover the earth with little colonies, demonstrating that simplicity of living plus high thinking lead to the greatest happiness!"

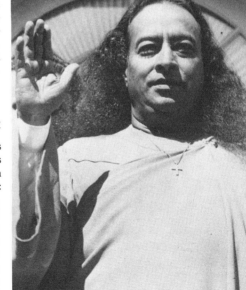

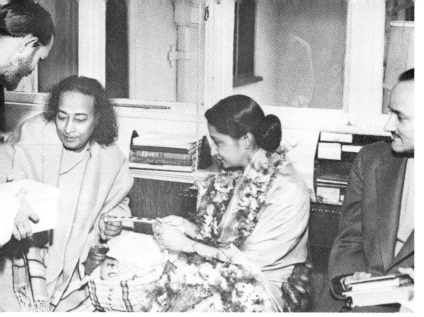

23

I present a box of Indian savories to Master for his guests on the occasion of India's Ambassador and his wife's visit to Mt. Washington.

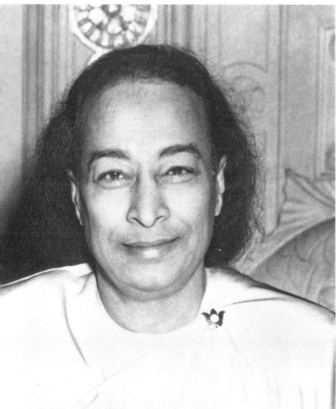

24

"I love you always, through endless cycles of time, unconditionally, without any desire except for *your* happiness, forever, in God!"

17

Mt. Washington Estates

MT. WASHINGTON, in the Highland Park district of Los Angeles, rises above that vast city like some guardian angel. At the mountaintop the sound of traffic through the busy streets below is hushed to a quiet hum. Though *in* the world, it seems a place not wholly *of* the world.

Atop Mt. Washington is located the international headquarters of Self-Realization Fellowship.

At the turn of the century, Mt. Washington Estates, as this property is known, was a fashionable hotel. The "city of angels" was much smaller then: some 100,000 inhabitants. In time, the city's inexorable engulfment of its surrounding orchards and farmland induced Mt. Washington's fashionable clientele to seek their recreation farther afield. Mt. Washington Estates fell on hard times. The busy world paid court to Mt. Washington no longer.

Unlike most once-fashionable resorts, however, pathetic in their memories of a heyday forever vanished, Mt. Washington's erstwhile glory was but the prelude to a far more glorious role.

Around the turn of the century, at the time when Mt. Washington had attained the height of its popularity as a resort, there was a young boy in India who, during periods of ecstatic meditation, caught glimpses of a mysterious mountaintop monastery in a distant land, visions concerning the mission that, he knew, he was meant someday to fulfill. Mukunda Lal Ghosh, later known to the world as Paramhansa Yogananda, was the son of a senior executive in the Bengal-Nagpur Railway; as such, he faced the prospect of wealth and high worldly position when he grew up. But it was not this world that attracted him. From earliest childhood he had longed for God as intensely as others long for human love or for worldly recognition.

Soon after graduation from high school, Mukunda met his guru,* the great Swami Sri Yukteswar of Serampore, Bengal. At the feet of this great master he attained, in the amazingly short space of six months, the high state of *samadhi,†* or unconditioned oneness with God. His guru kept him in the *ashram§* another nine and a half years, while he trained him for his mission of yoga dissemination in the West. "The West," Sri Yukteswar explained, "is high in material attainments, but lacking in spiritual understanding. It is God's will that you play a role in teaching mankind the value of balancing the material with an inner, spiritual life."

---

*Spiritual teacher. The word *guru* is often applied, broadly, to any venerated teacher. On the spiritual path, however, it refers to the *sadguru*, or *true* teacher—that enlightened sage who has been commissioned by God to lead the spiritually fit seeker out of darkness, and into the experience of Supreme Truth. While the seeker may have many lesser teachers, it is written that he can have only one such divinely appointed *guru*.

†*Samadhi* (cosmic consciousness) is the state of infinite awareness that comes to the yogi once the hypnosis of ego has been broken. Christian saints have sometimes described this state as "mystical marriage," for in it the soul merges into God and becomes one with Him.

§A place of retirement from worldly life for the purpose of pursuing spiritual practices.

In 1917, Mukunda, now a monk with the name Swami Yogananda, took the first outward step toward the fulfillment of his mission by founding a small school for boys in the village of Dihika, Bengal. In 1918 the Maharaja of Kasimbazar graciously gave him permission to transfer this fast-growing school to the Kasimbazar palace in Ranchi, Bihar. Here the school flourished. An institution offering education in the divine art of living along with the standard curriculum made an instant appeal to parents and children alike. In the first year, enrollment applications reached two thousand—far more than the existing facilities could absorb. By the end of two years, the young yogi-headmaster's educational theories were already beginning to have a serious impact on other educators.

Dear as Yogananda's Ranchi school was to him, however, there was another, broader mission for which the Lord was even now preparing him. In 1920 the youthful yogi had a vision: Thousands of Americans passed before him. The time had come for him to begin his lifework in the West.

The very next day he received an invitation to speak as India's delegate to an International Congress of Religious Liberals, being held that year in Boston, Massachusetts.

In America he found many people hungry for India's teachings, and for the liberating techniques of yoga.

In 1923 he began a series of lectures and classes in major American cities. His success everywhere was extraordinary. Crowds flocked to him in unprecedented numbers, sometimes queuing up for blocks to get in. Unlike most other teachers from India, he never tried to impose his own country's cultural modes on Americans, but sought rather to show Americans how to spiritualize *their own* culture. Dynamically, and with contagious joy, he set out to persuade minds steeped in the virtues of "down-to-earth practicality" that the most practical course of all is to seek God.

During his transcontinental tour in 1924, many would have been thrilled for Swami Yogananda to make his home in their cities. But to every such invitation he replied, "My soul calls me to Los Angeles." Years later, a guest at Mt. Washington asked him, "Which do you consider the most spiritual place in America?" "I have always considered Los Angeles the Benares* of America," the Master replied.

---

*Benares, or Varanasi, the holiest city of the Hindus.

To Los Angeles he came. People flocked to his lectures in unprecedented numbers even for that city, noted as it is for its fascination with matters spiritual. Weeks passed in unceasing public service. And then he informed his delighted students that he planned to establish his headquarters there.

In January, 1925, he was out driving one day with two or three students. They drove up winding Mt. Washington Drive. As they passed Mt. Washington Estates the Master cried out, "Stop the car!"

"You can't go in there," his companions protested. "That's private property!"

But Yogananda, not to be dissuaded, entered the spacious grounds and strolled about them in silence. At last, holding onto the railing above the tennis courts, he exclaimed quietly, "This place feels like home!"

When I came to the Master in 1948, Mt. Washington Estates was a monastery. At first, however, he planned to make it a "how-to-live" school similar to his well-known institution in India. For his hopes for spiritualizing the West rested on all-round education for the young. But soon he realized that his educational dreams were premature for this country. First, the grown-ups would have to be converted to his ideals; only then would there be properly trained teachers, and enough parents willing to send their children to his schools. Soon, therefore, Mt. Washington became a residential center for adults desirous of devoting their lives to God.

By 1935 the work was firmly established and flourishing. This was the year that Yogananda's guru, Swami Sri Yukteswar, summoned him back to India. The now-famous disciple spent a year there traveling about, addressing large audiences.

During that year Sri Yukteswar bestowed on his beloved disciple the highest of India's spiritual titles, *Paramhansa*.

In 1936, Yogananda returned to Mt. Washington.

One of the aims of his work had been, as he put it, "To spread a spirit of brotherhood among all people, and to aid in establishing, in many countries, self-sustaining colonies for plain living and high thinking." It was to the establishment of such a "world-brotherhood colony" that he now turned his energies.

The problem to which he addressed himself was similar to that which had first inspired his interest in child education. "Environment," he used to say, "is stronger than will power." The environment in which a child lives determines to a great extent his attitudes and behavior after he grows up. The environment an adult lives in, similarly, can make all the difference between success and failure in his efforts to transform old, unwanted habits. Paramhansaji urged people to live in harmonious environments, if possible. Most modern environments, alas, even when outwardly harmonious, are not spiritually uplifting.

The solution he arrived at was to provide places where family, friends, job, and general environment all would conduce to spiritual development. In the early nineteen-forties he set himself to found one such community.

Encinitas was the site he chose for this project. Here he began accepting families. In lecture after lecture in the churches he urged people to combine their meditative efforts with the simpler, freer lifestyle of a spiritual community. Though it was not possible for him to complete this project during his lifetime, his thought-force was, as he put it, "in the ether." It would find objective fulfillment in its own time.

In 1946 *Autobiography of a Yogi* was published. Its appearance marked the beginning of the last chapter of his life: the completion of his major literary works, and the arrival of a veritable flood of new disciples.

It was on March 7, 1952, that he left his body. It had been an incredibly fruitful life. By the time it ended, SRF centers flourished in many countries. Yogananda's disciples around the world numbered many tens of thousands. He had opened the West to India's teachings in a way that no other teacher has ever succeeded in doing. This was the first time that a great master from India had spent the greater part of his life in the West. It is largely as a result of his teaching and radiant personal example that there has been, in recent decades, such widespread and growing interest in India's spiritual teachings.

The headquarters for this vast movement is still, as it was during his lifetime, Mt. Washington Estates. Here it was that my own life of discipleship began.

18

First Impressions

MY FIRST GLIMPSE of Mt. Washington Estates was of tall palm trees that lined the entrance driveway on either side, waving gently in the slight breeze as though to extend a kindly greeting: "Welcome!" they seemed to murmur. "Welcome home!"

Norman showed me about the spacious grounds. We then went and stood quietly above two tennis courts, which, Norman said, were used now for gentler, more *yogic* forms of exercise. In silence we gazed out over the city far below us.

Yes, I reflected, this *was* home! For how many years had I wandered. I had begun to wonder if I belonged *anywhere*. But now, suddenly, I knew that I did belong: *right here* in this ashram; *here* with my guru; *here*, with his spiritual family! Gazing about me, I breathed deeply the peace that permeated this holy place.

Norman stood by my side, wordlessly sharing my elation. After a time we both faced the opposite direction, and looked up across an attractive lawn towards the large main building. Calmly self-contained, it seemed suggestive of an almost patrician benignity.

"Master's rooms are those on the top floor to the right," Norman said, pointing to a series of third-storey windows at the eastern end of the building.

He led me into a spacious lobby, simply and tastefully furnished. We passed through a door at the eastern end into three rooms that had been converted into a print shop. Proceeding towards the back of the building, we crossed over a narrow bridge that overlooked a small interior garden, and entered the main office. From here, Norman explained to me, books, printed lessons, and a continous stream of correspondence went out to yoga students around the world.

We re-entered the lobby at the western end. Here, large, sliding doors opened into a chapel. I was impressed by the tasteful simplicity of my new home. Everything looked restful, modest, harmonious.

"Come," said Norman, "let me show you our rooms. You've been assigned the one next to mine."

We left by a downstairs exit and, proceeding down the front driveway, arrived at a cottage about fifty feet from the main building, set picturesquely amid spreading trees, fragrant flowers, and succulents. I was charmed with the unassuming simplicity of this little outbuilding. Here, Norman explained, the hotel guests decades earlier had waited to take the cable car down to Marmion Way. Recently, he went on, smiling, the waiting room had been "renovated, after a manner of speaking," and divided into sleeping quarters for two. His was the larger of the new rooms. Why, I marveled, had we, young neophytes that we were, been assigned such delightful quarters?

Understanding came quickly. As we entered the building, I tried to suppress a smile. Here, set so idyllically amid stately grounds, was a scene incongruously reminiscent of the hasty reconstruction that must have followed bombing raids during the war. Schoolboys, Norman explained, had done all the work. As I examined the consequences, I wondered whether the boys hadn't considered the windows and the window frames separate projects altogether. At any rate, the windows hung at odd angles, as though disdaining to have anything to do with mere *frames*. Months later, as if to atone for their stern aloofness, they extended a friendly invitation to the winds of winter to come in and make merry.

The walls, made of plasterboard, had been cut more or less according to whim. They did manage to touch the ceiling—shyly, I thought—here and there, but the gap between them and the floor was in no place less than two inches. The resulting periphery made a lair, conveniently dark, for spiders of every description.

But it was the floor that provided the *pièce de résistance.* It appeared to be composed of a cross between pumice and cement. This substance, I later learned, was the proud invention of Dr. Lloyd Kennell, the alternate minister at our church in San Diego. Dr. Kennell had boasted that his product would "outlast the Taj Mahal." But in fact it was already doing its best to prove the Biblical dictum, "Dust thou art." Every footstep displaced a part of this miracle substance, which rose in little clouds to settle everywhere: on clothes, books, furniture. . . .

Not that the room held any furniture, except for a hard wooden bed which, Norman assured me, improved one's posture. The small closet had no door to protect clothes against the ubiquitous dust. With Norman's help I found an old, discarded quilt in the basement storeroom. Folded double, it made an adequate mattress. I also located an old dressing table, wobbly on its own legs, but fairly steady when propped into a corner. Next I found a small table, which acquitted itself admirably when leaned against a wall. For a chair an orange crate was pressed into service. And a few days later I came upon a large, threadbare carpet in the storeroom. Though the pattern was barely discernable, this important addition helped to hold down the dust from the fast-disintegrating floor. In place of a closet door, further search through the storeroom yielded a strip of monk's cloth, two feet wide, which I used to cover part of the opening. (Now at least I didn't have to *see* the dust as it settled on my clothes!) A light bulb dangled precariously at the end of a long, rather frayed wire in the center of the room. The bathroom was in the main building, which was kept locked at night. It wasn't until a year later that I was given curtains for the windows.

It no longer mystified me why the older monks preferred living in the main building. But I was so utterly thrilled to be here in the ashram of my guru that these inconveniences only made me laugh delightedly.

I laughed often now. The pent-up agony of recent years found release in wave after fresh wave of happiness. Everything I had always longed for seemed mine now, in my new way of life.

And yet, thrilled as I was, my mind importuned me with innumerable questions. My heart and soul were converted indeed, but my intellect lagged far behind. Reincarnation, karma, superconsciousness, divine ecstasy, the astral world, masters, gurus, breathing exercises, vegetarianism, health foods, *sabikalpa* and *nirbikalpa* samadhi, Christ Consciousness— huff! puff! For me these were all new and staggering concepts.

I worked on the grounds with Norman and an older monk named Jean, gardening, plastering, and doing whatever odd jobs were required.

The most attractive feature of my new quarters was a small basement, reached by a narrow set of steps at the far end of the room. It was ideal for a meditation room.

My first evening at Mt. Washington, Rev. Bernard, the disciple I'd met in Master's interview room at the Hollywood church, visited me in my room. He taught me an ancient yoga technique of concentration, and added some general counsel.

"When you aren't practicing this technique, try keeping your mind focused at the point between the eyebrows. This is the Christ center, the seat of spiritual vision."

"Would it help," I asked him, "if I kept my mind focused there all day long as well?"

"Very much! When Master lived in his guru's ashram he practiced keeping his mind fixed there all the time.

"Through concentration on this spiritual eye, the consciousness gradually takes on the quality of divine light. That is what Jesus meant when he said, 'If thine eye be single, thy whole body shall be full of light.' "*

After Bernard left me, I sat for a while practicing the techniques I had learned. Later on I went out and stood above the tennis courts again. I gazed out this time over a vast carpet of twinkling lights. How lovely in the night was this huge, bustling city! But electricity, I reminded myself, lights only the pathways of this world. The divine luminescence lights pathways to Infinity.

"Lord," I prayed, "though I stumble countless times, I will never cease seeking Thee. Lead my footsteps ever onward toward Thy infinite light!"

---

*Matthew 6:22.

19

The First Days
Of A Neophyte

THE DAILY ROUTINE at Mt. Washington was fairly individual. Freedom was given us, as it is in most Indian ashrams, for private spiritual practice. We met regularly for work and meals, and held occasional evening classes in the SRF printed lessons, following the classes with group meditation.

Soon I was looking forward to my times for meditation as eagerly as the worldly man looks forward to an evening's partying. Never had I dreamed there could be such a wealth of enjoyment within my own self!

Sundays we attended morning and evening services in our Hollywood church.

The church I found charming in its simplicity. Niches on either side of the sanctuary contained figurines depicting various leaders in the great world religions. Paramhansa Yogananda had named this a "Church of All Religions." Seats for about 115 people faced the small stage from which services were conducted. Along the back wall of the stage was an altar containing five niches, each with a picture of one of our line of gurus: Babaji, Lahiri Mahasaya, Swami Sri Yukteswar, Paramhansa Yogananda, and Jesus Christ.

Bernard, who was to conduct the service the first Sunday after my arrival, showed me around beforehand. "Why," I asked him, "is the picture of Jesus Christ on our altar, too? Surely *he* isn't in our line of gurus."

Bernard smiled. "Master has told us it was Jesus himself who appeared to Babaji, and asked him to send this teaching of Self-Realization to the West. 'My followers,' Jesus asserted, 'have forgotten the art of divine, *inner* communion. Outwardly they do good works, but they have lost sight of the most important of my teachings, to "seek the kingdom of God first." '*

"The work he sent through Master to the West is helping people commune inwardly with God."

"Tell me," I said, hesitating before taking this philosophical plunge, "why do we have pictures on our altar at all? If the state of consciousness we're seeking is inside, doesn't it hinder our development to have our attention diverted outwardly, to individuals?"

"No," Bernard replied. "You see, our masters *have* that state of consciousness. For us, it is difficult even to visualize such a state! By attuning ourselves to them, we begin to sense what it is they have, and to develop that same consciousness in ourselves. This is what is meant in the Bible by the words, 'As many as received him, to them gave he power to become the sons of God.'† One might say that *attunement* is the essence of discipleship."

The day of our first meeting on September 12th, Master returned to Encinitas. I didn't see him until two weeks later, when he was scheduled to preach again at Hollywood Church.

The church that day was divinely peaceful. As we entered, music

---

*Matthew 6:33

†John 1:12.

was sounding on the organ.

At last the curtains parted, and there stood Master, in his eyes a deep, penetrating gaze that seemed to bestow on each one present a special blessing.

He led us in chanting and meditation, then gave a brief interpretation of selected passages from the Bible and the *Bhagavad Gita*. His sermon followed—an altogether delightful blend of wit, devotional inspiration, and wisdom. Yogananda wore his wisdom without the slightest affectation, like a comfortable old jacket that one has been wearing for years.

"Behind every rosebush of pleasure," he cautioned us, "hides a rattlesnake of pain." He went on to urge us to seek our "pleasures" in God, and to ignore the fickle promises of this world.

"There are two kinds of poor people," he remarked—"those who wear cloth rags, and those who, though traveling in limousines, wear spiritual rags of selfishness and indifference to God. It is better to be poor physically, and have God in your heart, than to be materially rich without Him."

"Never say that you are a sinner," he went on to tell us. "You are a child of God! Gold, though covered over with mud for centuries, remains gold. Even so, the pure gold of the soul, though covered for eons of time with the mud of delusion, remains forever pure 'gold.' To call yourself a sinner is to identify yourself with your sins, instead of trying to overcome them. To call yourself a sinner is the greatest sin before God!"

Following the sermon, Bernard made a few announcements. He concluded by recommending *Autobiography of a Yogi* to newcomers. At this point Master interrupted him to say, "Many are coming from afar after reading the book. One recently read it in New York, and—Walter, please stand up."

I glanced around to see who this "Walter" might be who, like me, had read the book recently in New York. There was no one standing. Turning back to Master, I found him smiling at me! *Walter?!* "Ah, well," I thought philosophically, "a rose by any other name . . ." Self-consciously I rose to my feet.

"Walter read the book in New York," Master continued affectionately, "and left everything to come here. Now he has become one of us."

Members, lay and renunciate alike, smiled at me in blessing.

"Walter" was the name Master called me ever thereafter. No one else used this name, until, after Master's earthly passing, I longed for

every possible reminder of those precious years with him. I then asked
my brothers and sisters on the path to call me by that name.

Master spent the next few days at Mt. Washington.

A few days before Master's return, Norman had talked me into
joining him in the "Grape Cure," a diet of nothing but grapes and
grape juice. A few weeks of this cure would, Norman assured me,
purify my body, and help me to make rapid progress in the spiritual
life. Master saw us that Monday morning.

"Devotion is the greatest purifier," he remarked, smiling.

"Is it your wish then, Sir, that we break this fast?"

"Well, I don't want you to break your wills, now that you have set
them this way. But your time would be better spent if you worked on
developing devotion. A pure heart is the way to God, not a pure
stomach!"

Master disciplined only those who accepted his discipline.
Otherwise he was the soul of consideration. I remember him
sometimes inquiring gently of new disciples to whom he'd offered
mild correction, "You don't mind my saying that, do you?"

One of the traits that impressed me about him most deeply, as I got
to know him, was his quality of universal respect. It was a respect born
of the deepest concern for others' welfare. The veriest stranger was,
I'm convinced, as dear to him as his own disciples were.

Debi Mukherjee, a young monk from India, told me of an example
he had seen of the universality of this love. Master had invited him out
for a drive one afternoon. They were on their way home near
sundown.

"Stop the car!" Master cried suddenly. They parked by the curb. He
got out and walked back several doors to a small, rather shoddy-
looking variety shop. There, to Debi's astonishment, he selected a
number of items, none of them useful. "What on earth can he want
with all that junk?" Debi marveled. At the front counter the owner, an
elderly woman, added up the price. When Master paid it, she burst
into tears.

"I very badly needed just this sum of money today!" she cried. "It's
near closing time, and I'd almost given up hope of getting it. Bless you,
Sir. God Himself must have sent you to me in my hour of need!"

Master's quiet smile alone betrayed his knowledge of her difficulty.
He offered no word of explanation. The purchases, as Debi had
suspected, served no practical purpose thereafter.

At first I found it a bit awkward living with a master who was, as I
soon discovered, conscious of my inmost thoughts and feelings. But I

became increasingly grateful, too, for his insight. For here at last, I realized, was one human being whose misunderstanding I need never fear. Master was my friend, ever quietly, firmly on my side, anxious only to help me toward the highest understanding, even when I erred.

Toward the end of September he invited me to Encinitas. There a small group of us meditated with him one evening. Sitting in his presence, the thought came to me, "No wonder the Indian Scriptures praise above all else the uplifting influence of a true guru!" Never, by my unaided efforts alone, could I have plunged into meditation so suddenly, or so deeply.

Soon thereafter Master invited me to a retreat he had at Twenty-Nine Palms.

20

Twenty-Nine Palms

"YOU MUST KEEP THIS PLACE a secret," Bernard warned me as we drove out to Twenty-Nine Palms. "With the rapid growth of the work, Master needs a place where he can go to concentrate on his writings."

The monks' retreat was a small cottage on some fifteen acres of land. A tall windmill creaked and clanked complainingly with every breeze, as it pumped water up from a well. A grove of blue-green smoke trees hid the cottage from the seldom-traveled sand road. Even with the windmill, which seemed determined to go public with news of how hard it was made to work, this seemed a perfect spot for seclusion and meditation. Over the coming years I was to spend many months in these tranquil surroundings.

Master's place was five miles up the road, and located in a more developed area.

My first stay at Twenty-Nine Palms was for a weekend. Shortly thereafter, Master asked Norman and me to build him a small swimming pool behind the house. Taking an occasional break from his writing, he would come out and work with us for fifteen minutes or so. Whenever he did so, I felt a deep blessing.

One hot day at noon Norman and I stood up from our digging and stretched, grateful that lunchtime had arrived. We enjoyed our work, but there was no denying that it was also tiring. Besides, we were famished. Briefly we surveyed the yawning pit at our feet.

"God, what a hole!" exclaimed Norman. We gazed out over the mounds of sand we'd deposited about the grounds with the wheelbarrow. The very sight of them, lumped there in mute testimony to our exertions, only reinforced our fatigue.

At that moment Master came out of doors.

"Those mounds don't look very attractive," he remarked. "I wonder if they couldn't be leveled out. Would one of you mind fetching a two-by-four?"

Armed with the board, we stood before him apprehensively and awaited further instructions.

"Each of you hold the two-by-four at one end," Master said. "Then—just come over to this mound here. Pull the sand back toward you by pressing down hard on the board, and moving it slowly back and forth between you."

Probably even this meager description suffices to convey some idea of how difficult the job was. By the time we'd leveled one mound, Norman and I were panting heavily. Well, we reflected, at least we'd demonstrated that the job could be done. Master now, his curiosity satisfied, would no doubt tell us to go and have our lunch.

"Very good," he commented approvingly. "I *thought* that method would work. Now then, why don't we try it just once more—on that mound over there?"

Adjusting our expectations accordingly, we started in a second time.

"Very good!" Master commented once again. Evidently not wishing to place obstacles in the way of the momentum we'd built up, he said, "Let's do just one more—this one over here."

And after that: "One more."

And then again: "Just one more."

I don't know how many mounds we leveled, but. . . . "Just one more," Master said again.

Suddenly, getting the joke at last, I stood up and laughed. Master smiled back at me.

"I was playing with you! Now—go and have your lunch."

Often, in his training of us, he would push our equanimity to the limit, to see which way we would break. If we rebelled, it meant we had failed the test. But if we responded with an extra spurt of energy, we found his tests immeasurably strengthening.

In the foregoing test, Master helped Norman and me to learn to resist the thought of fatigue. Curiously, I found I was actually *less* tired after leveling those mounds than I had been beforehand. "The greater the will," as Master often said, "the greater the flow of energy."

Shortly thereafter, Master began inviting us indoors after hours to listen to him while he dictated his writings. The truths I learned during those sessions were invaluable.

I was struck also by the sheer, dynamic courage with which he taught. Some people, I knew, would be tempted to tone down the power of his words, as if, in making them bland, to make them more popularly acceptable. But the hallmark of greatness is extraordinary energy. Such energy is always challenging.

Master, more than any other teacher I have ever met, was able to stir people, to shake them with the unexpected, to charm them with a sudden funny story, or startle them into alertness with some novel piece of information. Like Jesus, he spoke with the ring of truth.

Gradually, as weeks passed, I found my heart opening like a flower under the sunrays of his love.

"Visualize the guru," he said one evening, "at the point between the eyebrows, the Christ Center. Then try to feel his response in your heart. When you feel it, pray deeply, 'Introduce me to God.' "

As I meditated on him, I often felt a wave of peace or love descend over me, suffusing my entire being. Sometimes answers to questions came, and a clearer understanding of qualities that I was trying to develop, or to overcome. Sometimes, in a single meditation on Master, I would find myself freed of some delusion that had plagued me for months, perhaps even for years. On one such occasion, as I approached him afterward and knelt for his blessing, he commented softly, "Very good!"

After we'd dug the hole for the swimming pool, other monks came out to help construct the wood forms, and to pour the concrete. We poured by hand with the aid of a small cement mixer. I shoveled the sand; someone else added the gravel; others maneuvered wheelbarrows to the pouring sites. Twenty-three hours we labored, pausing only occasionally. But we chanted to God as we worked, and the hours passed joyously. At the end we were all smiling happily.

All of us, that is, but one. This man, after an hour or two of half-hearted labor, had grumbled, "I didn't come here to shovel *cement!*" Sitting down, he watched us for the remainder of the day, reminding us occasionally that this wasn't what the spiritual path was all about. Interestingly, at the end of that long day he alone felt exhausted.

The subject of this disciple's unwillingness came up a few months later in a discussion with Master. "He told me," I remarked, "that he can't obey you implicitly, Sir, because he feels he must develop his own free will."

"But his will is not free," Master replied, "so long as it is bound by moods and desires. I don't *ask* anyone to follow me, but those who have done so have found true freedom.

"Sister," he continued, using the name by which he always referred to Sister Gyanamata, the elderly disciple whom I'd met on my first visit to Encinitas—"Sister used to run up and down all the time doing my bidding. One day a few of the others said to her, 'Why are you always doing what *he* says? You have your own will!' She answered, 'Well, but don't you think it's too late to change? And I must say, I have never been so happy in my life as I have been since coming here.' "

Master chuckled. "They never bothered her again!"

Already I, in my own little way, could endorse Sister Gyanamata's reply to those reluctant disciples. For the more I tuned my will to Master's, the happier I found I became.

"My will," Master said, "is only to do God's will." The proof of his statement lay in the fact that the more perfectly we followed his will, the freer we ourselves felt, in God.

As Christmas approached, my heart was singing with a happiness I had never before dreamed possible.

On the 24th we gathered in the chapel at ten in the morning for an all-day meditation, to invite the infinite Christ to be born anew in the "mangers" of our hearts.

On Christmas Day we exchanged gifts in the traditional manner. This day had, for its main feature, an afternoon banquet, after which Master addressed us. The sweetness of his speech so charmed me that I felt as though I were living in heaven.

The following day Master gave Kriya Yoga initiation. As I

approached him for his blessing, I opened my eyes to find him smiling at me blissfully.

On New Year's Eve we gathered for a midnight meditation, again led by Master, in the main chapel. At one point during the proceedings he softly beat a large gong, then gradually increased and decreased the volume, in waves. "Imagine this as the sound of *Aum*,"* he told us, "spreading outward to infinity."

At the same time, one hundred miles away in Encinitas, another group of disciples was meditating in the main room of the hermitage. They, too, heard the gong that Master was striking. One of the monks later told me, "It was as though someone were beating it in the hallway just outside the room."

The meditation that followed at Mt. Washington was enthralling.

Midnight came. Suddenly waves of noise swept upward from the city below, and inward from the surrounding neighborhood: factory whistles, car horns, shouts, as countless celebrants ushered in the New Year. A neighbor's door opened, and a voice screamed desperately into the night: "Happy New Year!"

How pathetic those festive tones, compared to the soul-joy we were experiencing in our little chapel! And how blessed, I reflected, how wonderfully happy I was to be in this holy place—at the feet of my divine guru! I prayed that the New Year would bring me an ever deepening awareness of God's love.

---

*The vibration by which the universe is manifested. *Aum* is the Holy Ghost of the Christian Trinity.

21

Paramhansa Yogananda

ON JANUARY 5TH, the disciples gathered at Mt. Washington to celebrate Paramhansa Yogananda's birthday. At a banquet he spoke of his longing to see an awakening of divine love throughout the world. "I never dreamt, during my first years of teaching in this country, that such a fellow-feeling in God's love would be possible here. It exists only because you have lived up to the ideals that I have cherished, and which I lived for in the company of my great guru."

Friendship in God, surely, was the key to our relationship with him. It implied no easy-going relationship, such as worldly people enjoy with one another, but rather demanded of us the utmost. The friendship our guru extended to us was to our souls. To reciprocate in kind meant to strive ever to meet him on that divine level. Those who clung to the desire for ego-gratification could not coax from him a compromise in the pure quality of his friendship for us. If a disciple flattered him, Master would gaze at him quietly as if to say, "I will not desecrate the love I bear you by accepting this level of communication." Always he held out to us the highest ideal to which each of us might aspire. Such perfect love imposes the most demanding of all disciplines, for it asks nothing less of the disciple, ultimately, than the total gift of himself to God.

The Indian Scriptures state that when the soul releases its hold on egoism, it merges into the ocean of Spirit and becomes one with it. While most of us loved Master from varying degrees of ego-consciousness, his love for us was without limit, cosmic. To ordinary human beings, such love is inconceivable. "I killed Yogananda long ago," he said. "No one dwells in this temple now but God." His love for us was God's love, manifested through his human form.

It always amazed me that one whose wisdom and power inspired so much awe in others could be at the same time so humbly respectful to everyone. I once saw Master chat with a group of Indians after a public performance in Pasadena. One man in the group was, as the saying goes, "feeling no pain." Affecting great familiarity in his drunkenness, he threw an arm around Master's shoulders and shouted playfully, as though the two of them were old drinking buddies. Debi, who was standing nearby, made some disparaging remark in Bengali.

"Don't," Master replied, shaking his head a little sternly. In his eyes this man, regardless of his temporary condition, deserved the respect due to a child of God.

In Ranchi, India, I was told a touching story dating back to Master's return there in 1935. It seems an anniversary banquet was planned at his school. Someone was needed to preside over the function and give it official standing. The name of Gurudas Bannerji, a prominent judge, was recommended. Widely esteemed, this man was, as everyone agreed, the best possible choice. Master went to invite him.

What was his surprise, then, when the judge coldly refused to come. He knew all about India's so-called "holy men," he said; he was looking at a typical example of them right before him. They were insincere, after people's money, a drain on the community. He had no time to speak for their worthless causes.

Master, though astonished at this reception, remained unruffled. As he often told us, "Praise cannot make me any better, nor blame

any worse. I am what I am before my conscience and God." After
hearing the judge out, he replied in a friendly tone, "Well, perhaps
you'll reconsider. We should be greatly honored if you would
come."

The principal of a local school agreed to preside in the judge's
stead. When everyone had assembled that evening for the banquet,
and the affair was about to begin, a car drove up. Out stepped the
caustic judge. Because Gurudas Bannerji was such a prominent figure
in those parts, the school principal readily offered up his own place
to him.

Following the banquet, there were several preliminary reports.
One dealt with the school's growth, and the number of students who
had gone on after graduation to become monks and religious
teachers. "If the present trend continues," the report read, "soon all
of India will be full of our teachers spreading the ancient wisdom of
our land."

It then came the judge's turn to speak. Rising, he said: "Today is
one of the happiest days of my life. This morning your Swami
Yogananda came to visit me. I felt great joy when I beheld him, but I
decided to test him to see whether he was really as good a man as he
looked. I addressed him as rudely as I knew how. Yet he remained so
calm, and answered me so kindly, that I tell you in all sincerity he
passed my test better than I would have dreamed possible. And I will
tell you something more: Never mind the numbers of your graduates
who are becoming monks. India has many monks. But if you can
produce even one such man as this, not your school only, nor only
our city, but our whole country will be glorified!"

Wonderful as Master's quality of universal respect was, it might
be supposed that it entailed at least one disadvantage: an inability to
see the funny side of what is often called the human comedy. The
supposition would be unwarranted. The truth is, I have never known
anyone with a keener sense of the ridiculous.

One day, in Chicago, a drunken stranger staggered up to him
and embraced him affectionately.

"Hello there, Jeshush Chrisht!"

Master smiled. Then, to give the man a taste of the infinitely better
"spirits" he himself enjoyed, he looked deeply into the man's eyes.

"Shay," the fellow cried thickly, "whad're *you* drink'n'?"

"It has a lot of kick in it!" Master replied, his eyes twinkling. The
man was sobered by this glance. "I left him wondering what had
happened!" Master told us later.

Even as a boy, the Master's magnetism was extraordinary. Dr. Nagendra Nath Das, a Calcutta physician and lifelong friend, visited Mt. Washington in July, 1950. He told us, "Wherever Paramhansaji went, even as a boy, he attracted people. His father, a high railway official, often gave us travel passes. No matter where we traveled, within minutes after we'd got down from the train a group of boys would have gathered about us."

Part of the basis for Master's amazing charisma was the fact that, seeing his infinite Beloved in all human beings, he also awakened in them an inchoate faith in their own goodness. With the impersonality of true greatness, he never accepted the thought from others that he was essentially any different from them.

Bernard, upon whom Master had been urging some difficult undertaking, remonstrated one day, "Well, Sir, *you* can do it. You're a *master*."

"And what do you think *made* me a master?" the guru demanded. "It was by *doing!* Don't cling to the thought of weakness if your desire is to become strong."

This was the relationship that Master sought ever to establish with us: a relationship wherein we realized with our entire being that we, too, were *That*.

22

Renunciation

M Y SUDDEN CONVERSION to this totally un-
heralded way of life had the effect on my earthly
family that a grenade might have if hurled
unexpectedly into someone's home during a
leisurely Sunday breakfast. My parents believed strongly in giving us
children the freedom to follow our own lights, but even so, their
concern for my happiness made them anything but indifferent to
what struck them as a sudden plunge into insanity.

Some weeks after my arrival at Mt. Washington, I received a letter
from Father Kernan, the associate minister at our Church of St.
James the Less in Scarsdale. Was I, he inquired sympathetically, in
some emotional or spiritual difficulty?

Sue and Bud Clewell, relatives in Westwood Village (a suburb of

Los Angeles), visited me with pleas that I not estrange myself from the family. My brother Bob wrote from New York to suggest that I might like to join him in some housing-development scheme.

People who want to dedicate their lives to high ideals often encounter opposition from well-meaning friends and relatives. Indeed, between selfless idealism and worldliness there exists a fundamental incompatibility. The worldly person asks first of life, "What do *I* want?" The devotee asks only, "What does God want?"

The pathway of the heart is too narrow for both the ego and God to walk it together; one of them must step aside and make way for the other. Anything that binds us to a limited existence desecrates this divine image within us. Renunciation is no abject self-deprivation, but a glorious affirmation of the universe of joy that is our birthright.

In the Self-Realization Fellowship monasteries, Paramhansa Yogananda taught us boldly to claim our new identity as sons of God, rejecting all consciousness of worldly ties.

"Sir," I began one day, "my father . . ."

"You have no father!" Master peremptorily reminded me. "God is your Father."*

Nothing won Master's approval so much as the willingness to renounce all for God. But renunciation, to him, meant an inner act of the heart; outward symbols he viewed more tentatively, as potential distractions to sincerity. For this present age, prejudiced as it is against many aspects of the spiritual life, he counseled only moderate adoption of the outward symbols of renunciation. Perhaps he felt that more extreme austerities might attract too much attention to themselves, and thus feed the very ego which the renunciate was striving to overcome. "Make your heart a hermitage," he counseled us. It was not so much that he rejected outward forms; his concern was that we use them to *internalize* our devotion.

"Don't mix with others too closely," he recommended to us one evening. "The desire for outward companionship is a reflection of

---

*"One said unto him, Behold, thy mother and thy brethren stand without, desiring to speak with thee. But he answered and said unto him that told him, Who is my mother? and who are my brethren? and he stretched forth his hand toward his disciples, and said, Behold my mother and my brethren! For whosoever shall do the will of my Father which is in heaven, the same is my brother, and sister, and mother." (Matthew 12:46-50.)

the soul's inward desire for companionship with God. But the more you seek to satisfy that desire outwardly, the more you will lose touch with the inner, divine Companion, and the more restless and dissatisfied you will become."

Frequently he held up to us examples of saints who had remained aloof even from fellow devotees. "Seclusion," he said, "is the price of greatness."

Disciples seeking help in overcoming delusion received loving encouragement and sympathetic counsel.

"If the sex drive were taken away from you," he told a group of monks one evening, "you would see that you had lost your greatest friend. You would lose all interest in life. Sex was given to make you strong. If a boxer were to fight only weaklings, he too, in time, would grow weak. It is by fighting strong men that he develops strength. The same is true in your struggle with the sex instinct. The more you master it, the more you will find yourself becoming a lion of happiness."

The three greatest human delusions, he used to say, are sex, wine (by which he meant intoxicants of all kinds), and money.

"Meditate," he urged us. "The more you taste God's joy within you, the less taste you will have for those mere masquerades of ecstasy."

Rejection of the world is only the negative side of devotion. Master's usual emphasis was positive. "Nothing can touch you," he told us, "if you inwardly love God." Nevertheless, there is a beauty in the act of utter self-offering to God that makes renunciation, even in its more limited, negative aspect, one of the most heroic and noble callings possible to man.

Bernard told me of one occasion when a visitor from India came to see Paramhansa Yogananda. The man was received by Sister Gyanamata, and had the poor grace to treat her condescendingly—as though, in serving her guru, she were only Master's servant. Later, inspired by his interview with Master, he apologized to her.

"In India," he said, "we are taught to respect all women as wives and mothers. Forgive me, please, that I failed to pay you that respect earlier." Smilingly he concluded, "I offer it to you now."

Sister Gyanamata, in her usual impersonal manner, replied, "At least half the people in the world are women. Most of them sooner or later become mothers. There is nothing in either fact that merits any special respect. But you may, if you wish, pay respect to the fact that in this life I have become a renunciate."

The visitor could only bow. For renunciation of egoic desires and attachments is, ultimately, the stepping stone for all people, whether married or single, to rediscovery of that divine image within, which alone gives man importance in the greater scheme of things.

23

God Protects His Devotees

NORMAN ENTERED the dining room one day at lunchtime looking stunned.

"This morning," he announced shakily, "I was driving the big flat-bed truck down Mt. Washington. As I came to the steepest part of the hill, I stepped on the brake to slow down for that hairpin turn at the bottom, but my foot went right to the floor! I pumped frantically; nothing happened. By this time the truck was going so fast I couldn't shift down. In moments I knew I'd be hurtling to my death over the edge of that steep embankment. Desperately I prayed to Master: 'Is this what you want?'

"Suddenly the truck slowed to a complete stop! The brakes still weren't working, but I was able to park safely in gear and curb the front wheel.

"What a blessing," Norman concluded, "to have a God-realized master for a guru!"

We often found that we had only to call Master mentally for misfortune to be speedily averted.

Once, Joe Carbone and Henry Schaufelberger (now Brothers Bimalananda and Anandamoy) were plastering the lotus tower that forms the archway entrance to the SRF church grounds in Hollywood. Joe was mixing and carrying the plaster. Henry, at a height of about twenty feet, was troweling it onto the wall. The ladder Joe was using was set at too steep an angle. On one climb, as he reached up to grasp the top rung, he missed it. The heavy hod on his shoulder began pulling him backward; he could no longer grasp the rung with either hand. A twenty-foot drop with all that weight on his shoulder might very well have killed him. Realizing that it was too late to save himself, Joe thought urgently of Master, and chanted, "Om!"

Both men later testified as to what happened next. As Joe was chanting, some invisible force pushed him slowly back upright. A moment later he was able to grasp the rung again. Gasping with relief, he completed his climb.

In the almost thirty years that I have been on this path, I cannot recall to mind a single instance where a disciple of Paramhansa Yogananda has failed to find protection in time of real need. Considering the length of time involved, and the thousands of disciples I have known during this period, this is quite an amazing record.

The most striking of these cases occurred among those whose lives were placed unreservedly in the guru's care. Dr. Lewis told of an episode similar to Norman's, when, on a cold winter night in Massachusetts, he had been out driving. With him were two fellow disciples. As they approached a narrow bridge, they found their way blocked by another car. A crash seemed inevitable.

"At that moment," Dr. Lewis said, "we felt as if a giant hand were pressing down on the hood of the car. We slowed instantly to a stop."

Señor J. M. Cuaron, the leader of the SRF center in Mexico City, related the following incident to me.

"I was badly in need of a job, but for a long time could find none anywhere. Then one day an excellent offer came from a company in Matamoros. Taking that job would mean moving away from Mexico City. I therefore wrote Master to request his permission to put the center in someone else's charge. I was sure Master would congratulate me on my good luck. Imagine my surprise, then, when he replied by telegram: 'No. Absolutely not. Under no circumstances whatever accept that job.' I'll admit I was a bit upset. But even so, I obeyed him.

"One month later the news came out in the papers: The company that had offered me that job was exposed for fraud. Its officers were sent to prison, including the man who had taken the post I'd been offered. He hadn't been aware of the firm's dishonesty, just as I wouldn't have been. But because of the position he held, he was imprisoned. It was only by Master's grace that I was spared that calamity!"

Tests there must be in life, of course. They come especially on the spiritual path, for if devotees are to escape the coils of *maya* (delusion), they must be taught the lessons they need to develop in wisdom. Tests came indeed, but outright misfortune Master spared us. Where a test was not required for our growth, Master often removed it from our path altogether.

In 1955, in Switzerland on a lecture tour, I met a Czechoslovakian lady who told me a story concerning Professor Novicky, the late leader of a small SRF group in Prague.

"One day," she said, "after Yogananda's passing, a stranger came to Professor Novicky and requested instruction in yoga. The professor normally kept his spiritual activities a secret, so as not to expose himself to persecution. But if this man was a genuine seeker, he would want to help him. Yet if he was a government spy, any admission of interest in yoga might result in a prison sentence. Our friend prayed for guidance. Suddenly, standing behind the self-proclaimed 'devotee,' Paramhansa Yogananda appeared. Slowly the Master shook his head, then vanished. Professor Novicky told the man he had come to the wrong place for information. Sometime later, he learned that the man was indeed a spy.

"I am free to tell this story now," my informant continued. "The professor died recently, of natural causes."

Death must, of course, come to everyone sooner or later. But I have been struck by its beauty and dignity when it has visited disciples of the path.

A member of our Hollywood church died of a stroke. His wife later told me, "In his final moments, my husband whispered to me lovingly, 'Don't feel badly, dear. I am so happy! And I see bright light all around me.' "

Another church member exclaimed at death. "Swamiji is here!" Her face radiant, she smiled blissfully.

And Sister Gyanamata's last words were, "Such joy! Too much joy! Too much joy!"

Disciples who have died of cancer or other painful diseases have gone peacefully, with a smile on their lips.

People often point to the sufferings of humanity as proof either that God doesn't exist, or that He doesn't care for His human children. Paramhansa Yogananda's answer to that charge was that people don't care enough about God to tune in to His help. Indeed, by their indifference they create the very problems which, later, they lay accusingly at His door. If in daylight one moves about with closed eyes, he may bump against something and hurt himself. By closing one's eyes to light, one creates his own darkness. By closing one's heart to love, one creates his own fear, hatred, or apathy. By closing one's soul to joy, one creates his own misery.

In case after case I have seen fulfilled Yogananda's promise that faithful devotees of his path would be protected. "For those who stay in tune to the end," he added, "I, or one of the other masters, will be there to usher them into the divine kingdom." Truly, the words of the great Swami Shankaracharya have found justification in Paramhansa Yogananda's life: "No known comparison exists in the three worlds for a true guru."

24

True Teaching
Is Individual

MASTER WAS, to each one of us, like a flawless mirror. He held up to our inner gaze, not his opinions of us, but the subtle reactions of our own higher natures. His perfect self-transcendence never ceased to amaze me. In another person's company he actually, in a sense, *became* that person. I don't mean that in our company he assumed our weaknesses, our pettiness, our moods of anger or despondency. What he showed us, rather, was the silent watcher deep within our own selves.

In his training of us his teaching was individual also. It was not that he *altered* basic teachings to suit our personal needs. It was his emphasis, rather, that varied. To some he stressed attitudes of service; to others, deep inwardness. To one he emphasized the need for greater joy; to another, for less levity.

In our work, one might have expected him to honor that basic principle of every well-run institution: "Make the best use of individual talent." But to Master this practice would have meant *using* his disciples. His true concern, always, was for our spiritual needs. Sometimes he would actually take us away from some important assignment—one, perhaps, for which no one else could be found—simply to help us spiritually. Sometimes, too, he placed people in positions for which they weren't qualified, with a view to prompting them, in their struggle to meet his expectations, to develop needed spiritual qualities. Or he would not place people in positions for which they were eminently qualified, simply because they no longer needed those particular experiences to grow spiritually. Sister Gyanamata, for example, his most advanced woman disciple, and a person of deep wisdom, could have rendered enormous assistance by lecturing, teaching, and writing. But Master never asked her to serve in any such role. That kind of work simply wasn't necessary for her spiritual growth.

My own deep-seated desire had always been to share joy with others. Having suffered spiritually myself, I felt deeply the spiritual sufferings of others, and longed to do all I could to help assuage their sufferings. Master responded to this deep inner longing of mine, and trained me from the beginning for public service. He put me into office work, answering letters, and asked me to write articles for our bimonthly magazine.

One day he instructed me to stand outside the church after Sunday morning services and shake hands with people as they left. In his lessons he states that people exchange magnetism when shaking hands. Thus, what Master wanted me to do was not merely greet people, but act as his channel of blessings to others. The first time I tried it, I felt so drained of energy I actually became dizzy. I suppose what happened was that people unconsciously drew from me, in the consciousness that I was serving as Master's representative.

"Master," I said, "I'm not ready for this job!"

"That is because you are thinking of yourself," he replied. "Think of God, and you will find *His* energy flowing through you."

His suggestion worked. By holding to the thought of God, I discovered that I felt actually more uplifted after shaking hands with the congregation than beforehand.

"When this 'I' shall die," Master wrote once in a rhymed couplet, "then shall I know who am I."

One of my jobs was to send weekly advertisements of church services to the newspapers. Master had been lecturing fortnightly in our San Diego church. Of recent months, however, he had taken to going there only occasionally. The church members, ever anxious to see him, were instructed to check the church page of the *San Diego Union* every Saturday. Whenever Master came, the church was full to overflowing.

One week in May I was instructed to send in the announcement that Master, after a two months absence, would appear there the following Sunday. I smiled. How delighted the congregation would be!

Saturday morning Bernard came to my room with horrifying news. "Master can't go to San Diego after all. He wants you to speak in his stead."

"*Me!* But . . . but I've never lectured before in my life!"

"He also wants you to give a Kriya Yoga initiation afterwards."

"Oh, those poor people!"

"You'll only have to initiate one of them," Bernard consoled me. "Here's money for the bus."

With sinking heart I drove down to San Diego. Through closed curtains Sunday morning I heard the murmurs of a large and eagerly waiting crowd.

The dreaded moment arrived. I stood up. The curtains parted. My worst fears were realized: The church was completely packed. People were standing in the aisles. Others craned their necks to peer in through the windows. I could feel their shock as an almost physical wave. Instead of their long-awaited guru, here facing them was an unknown and rather lost-looking boy of twenty-two. Sorry for them in their disappointment, I forgot the awkwardness of my own position. If everyone there had walked out, I would have understood. But regular meditation, I suppose, had made them gracious. No one left.

The Kriya initiation that afternoon frightened me even more than the service had. Michelle Evans, the lady I initiated, looked as terrified as I was—infected, as she later admitted, by my own fear. But Master's blessings, powerfully felt, soon dispelled all anxiety. The ceremony went smoothly. I returned to Mt. Washington that afternoon bowed, perhaps, but unbloodied.

Later, Master received compliments on my lecture. "Most of all," he reported, pleased, "they liked your humility." I reflected that, under the circumstances, humility had been virtually unavoidable!

From this time onward, Master had me lecture regularly in the churches. He referred to me publicly as "Reverend Walter," though the actual formalities of ordination weren't completed until a year later.

"Your desire to be happy," he often told us, "must include others' happiness." I had always known in my heart that I would be called upon someday to serve others through teaching and lecturing. But whether out of the humility that Master sometimes praised in me, or from darker motives of unwillingness, it was, I'm afraid, not a few years before I could bring myself to believe that my lectures really did anyone any good.

Master, however, made it clear that he expected me to take this responsibility seriously. "Sir," I once pleaded with him, "I don't want to be a lecturer!"

"You'd better learn to like it," he replied pleasantly. "That is what you will have to do."

25

Work Vs. Meditation

"**M**ASTER ONCE TAUGHT ME a good lesson on the attitude we should hold toward our work." Mrs. Vera Brown (now Meera Mata), an advanced older disciple whom Master had made responsible for training some of the newer ones, was sharing with me a few of her experiences with our guru.

" 'You work too hard,' Master told me one day. 'You *must* work less. If you don't, you will ruin your health.'

" 'Very well,' I thought, 'I'll try not doing so much.'

"Two or three days later, much to my surprise, Master gave me *more* work to do!"

Mrs. Brown's eyes twinkled. " 'Okay, Master,' I thought, 'you must know what you're doing.' I took on my new duties. But all the time I kept wondering, 'How am I going to reconcile all this extra work with his instructions to me to work *less?*'

"Well, a couple of days after that Master again told me, sternly this time, 'You *must not* work so hard. In this lifetime you've done enough work for several incarnations.'

"What was I to do? Again I tried cutting down my activities, only to find Master, after two or three days, giving me more work than ever!

"We repeated this little act several times. Every time Master told me to work *less,* he soon added duties that forced me to work *more.* I figured he must know what he was doing, and that it was up to me to try and understand what that was.

"Well, finally one day I looked at Master. 'Sir,' I said, 'instead of our using the word, *work,* in our life here, why don't we substitute the word, *service?*'

"Master laughed. 'It has been a good show,' he said. 'All your life you've been thinking, *work! work! work!* That very thought was exhausting you. But just see how differently you feel when you think of work as a divine service! When you act to please God you can do *twice* as much, and never feel tired!' "

Mrs. Brown, whose frail body never seemed to run out of energy no matter how much she did, laughed merrily. "You see, the very thought of pleasing God fills us with *His* energy. Master tells us it's our unwillingness that cuts off that flow of energy."

The spiritual path would, one suspects, be relatively easy to understand if it involved only meditation, ecstatic visions, and blissful expansions of consciousness. Why, one asks, must it be complicated by mundane activities like ditch digging and letter writing and cleaning up kitchens? One may sympathize, on one level at least, with that reluctant disciple the day we completed the swimming pool at Twenty-Nine Palms who grumbled, "I didn't come here to pour *cement!*" Many a sincere devotee, too, has probably wondered what pouring cement (or digging ditches, or writing letters, or cleaning up kitchens) has to do with finding God.

The answer is, quite simply: *nothing!* Not in itself, anyway. The purpose of spiritual work is not really to do things for God, but rather to do the most important thing of all for ourselves: to purify our own hearts. Work, on the spiritual path, is a means of helping one to channel his energies constantly, *dynamically,* toward God.

"Make every minute count," Master said. "The minutes are more important than the years." People who put their whole concentration into working for God find they can also meditate more deeply.

"When you work for God, not self," Master told us one day, "that is just as good as meditation. Then work helps your meditation, and meditation helps your work. You need the balance. With only meditation you become lazy, and the senses become strong. With only work, the mind becomes restless, and you forget God."

Master taught us not only to offer our work moment by moment to God, but also to see God acting through us as the real Doer. To see God as the Doer means recognizing that it is *His* energy and inspiration by which we live. It means not taking personal credit for anything we do. This attitude keeps one humble, and also vastly increases one's powers of accomplishment.

Master urged us always to keep a positive outlook, to affirm possibilities rather than weaken them with too many so-called "reasonable" objections.

I remember his greeting to me one day: "How are you, Walter?"

"Well," I began. . . .

"That's good!" he interposed promptly, nipping in the bud what he saw was only a mild case of "vapors."

Never supportive of us in our moods, he urged us to banish them firmly with vigorous, positive affirmations.

Moods weren't often my specific problem, but I remember one that ambushed me one day, and the helpful method I discovered for combatting it.

It was in February or March, 1949. Master had been away from Mt. Washington several weeks, and I hadn't seen him in all that time. I was beginning to feel his absence keenly. Finally he returned. The next day word was sent down to me to get someone to carry a five-gallon bottle of drinking water up to his kitchen. Eagerly I appropriated the job to myself. Arriving upstairs with the bottle, I could hear Master dictating a letter in his sitting room. Hoping to attract his attention, I rattled the bottle and made as much noise as I felt I decently could for a job that called for a minimum of tumult. Master paid no attention.

"He doesn't care that I miss him!" I thought, plunging suddenly into a violent depression. "I'm just a worker to him, not a disciple!" I rushed on to brood over the unfeeling nature of this world, where nobody really cares for anybody else. Moments later I made an abrupt about-face: "No, Master cares, but he sees I'm such a hopeless case that he might as well give up pouring water into a bottomless pit!'' On and on my mind churned. I tried reasoning with myself: "Look here, he's obviously busy. Why should he drop everything just for you?"

"Yeah?" retorted my recalcitrant mind. "I imagine he said, 'Look out, here comes that worthless disciple, Walter! Quick, let me dictate a letter as an excuse not to have to call him in here.' "

Clearly, reason wasn't going to pull me out of this mental whirlpool. Indeed, reason's tendency is to support any feeling that happens to be uppermost in the mind.

"Do you *like* being moody?" I demanded of my mental citizens.

"No!" came the chorus—unanimously, except for one or two grumblers in the background.

"Very well, then, boys, if reason won't do it, let's see if changing our level of consciousness will do the trick."

I went down to my meditation "cave," and there plunged my mind deeply at the Christ Center between the eyebrows. Five minutes was all it took. By the end of that time my mood was so positive that I no longer needed to affirm anything. "But *of course* he's busy!" I thought. "Hasn't he often told us that our real communion with him is *inside*, in meditation? And what if all his disciples tried selfishly to take up his time? He wouldn't have any time left over to complete his writings, which will help thousands."

Master's help was available to anyone who called to him mentally in meditation. Here he was the guide, ever subtly inspiring us, according to the measure of our receptivity, to make the right kind of spiritual effort. Sometimes, too, when we met him during the couse of the day, he would admonish us on some point concerning our meditations. Indeed, he watched over us in all ways. It never ceased to amaze me that, with so many disciples to look after, he could be so perfectly aware of each of our needs.

"I go through your souls every day," he told us. "If I see something in you that needs correcting, I tell you about it. Otherwise, I say nothing." On another occasion he said, "I have lived the lives of each one of you. Many times I go so deep at night into a person that when I wake up in the morning I think I *am* that person! It can be a terrible experience, if he happens to be someone full of moods and desires."

Master responded instantly to sincere love. One day, missing him intensely, I went down to see him in Encinitas where he was staying at the time. Shortly after my arrival he passed a group of us on his way back from a drive. Seeing me, he invited me to ride up with him to the hermitage. "I have missed you," he told me lovingly. How rare is it, I thought, for one's unexpressed feelings to be caught so sensitively.

26

The Ministry

BY JUNE, 1949, I was conducting midweek services more or less regularly. Soon I also gave occasional Sunday services. A problem for any new speaker is how to avoid nervousness. My own problem was accentuated by my youth. The average age of my listeners was about forty. I could count on their knowing a great deal more about most things than I did.

The solution I found was to imagine the worst audience response possible, and accept it. "It is all God's dream anyway," I reminded myself. Then I learned to see the people I was speaking to as manifestations of God. *Through* them, rather than by merely surviving the personal ordeal of appearing before them, I was being asked to serve Him.

At first I used to pray before every lecture, "Lord, inspire me to say what *You* want said." Later I learned to ask Him also, "Help me sense what this particular audience needs to hear through me." I learned in time to prepare minimally, if at all, for my lectures, for I found that an open mind enabled me to respond more sensitively to the unvoiced needs of my listeners. People began thanking me after my lectures for answering their specific questions, or for dealing with problems that had been weighing on their minds.

Master also gave me the following advice: "Before lecturing, meditate deeply. Then, holding that meditative calmness, think about what you intend to say. Write down your ideas. Include one or two funny stories; people are more receptive when they can enjoy a good laugh. Then finish with a story from the SRF lessons. After that, put the subject out of your mind. While speaking, keep mentally before you the salient points of your outline, but above all ask the Spirit to flow through you. In that way you will draw your inspiration from that inner Source, and will not speak from ego."

Most important of all to Master was the question of our attunement while lecturing, that we might share with our listeners not only our ideas, but our vibrations. Late one Thursday afternoon he spied Dr. Lewis out on the grounds in Encinitas, enjoying a stroll.

"Doctor, aren't you giving the service this evening? Then what are you doing roaming about? You should be meditating!"

In time I reached the point where I could actually *feel* a power flowing from my attunement with Master, and filling any room in which I might be lecturing. If anything I said touched my listeners, the credit was due to this power far more than to any words I uttered.

Master's own services were rich with inspiration. They conveyed none of the orphaned feeling that one encounters in many churches, of a God living distantly in some unimaginable heaven, or of a Jesus Christ who left no more vital testimony to his continuing reality than the printed words in the Bible. In Master's presence, divine truths came thrillingly alive, made vibrant with the immediacy of his own God-realization.

"You are a good salesman!" an American businessman exclaimed after one of his lectures. "That," Master replied, "is because I have sold myself on the truths I teach!"

Some of my most impressive memories of Master are of his public lectures. While they lacked the sweet intimacy of talks with the disciples at Mt. Washington, they rang with the spirit of a mission destined, he told us, to bring spiritual regeneration to the world.

I remember especially how affected I was by a talk he gave at a garden party in Beverly Hills. It was the most stirring lecture I have ever heard.

"This day," he thundered, punctuating every word, "marks the birth of a new era. My spoken words are registered in the ether, in the Spirit of God, and they shall move the West. . . . Self-Realizaion has come to unite all religions. . . . We must go on—not only those who are here, but thousands of youths must go North, South, East and West to cover the earth with little colonies, demonstrating that simplicity of living plus high thinking lead to the greatest happiness!"* I was moved to my core. It would not have surprised me had the heavens opened up and a host of angels come streaming out, eyes ablaze, to do his bidding. Deeply I vowed that day to do my utmost to make his words a reality.

Often during the years I was with Master he exhorted his audiences on the subject of this cherished dream of his : "world-brotherhood colonies," or spiritual cooperative communities—not monasteries, merely, but places where people in every stage of life could devote themselves to living the divine life.

"Gather together, those of you who share high ideals," Yogananda told his audiences. "Pool your resources. Buy land out in the country. A simple life will bring you inner freedom. Harmony with nature will bring you a happiness known to few city dwellers. In the company of other truth seekers it will be easier for you to meditate and think of God.

"What is the need for all the luxuries people surround themselves with? Most of what they have they are paying for on the installment plan. Their debts are a source of unending worry to them. Even people whose luxuries have been paid for are not free; attachment makes them slaves. They consider themselves freer for their possessions, but don't see how their possessions in turn possess them!"

He added: "The day will come when this colony idea will spread through the world like wildfire."

Master wanted to start a model world-brotherhood colony in Encinitas. He felt deeply the importance of this communitarian

---

*Self-Realization Magazine, November-December, 1949, p. 36.

dream; for years it formed the nucleus of all his plans for the work.

But alas, he encountered an obstacle that has stood in the way of every spiritual reform since the days of Buddha: human nature. Marriage has always tended to be something of a closed corporation. The economic depression of the Nineteen-Thirties had had the effect on a generation of Americans of heightening this tendency by increasing their desire for worldly security. "Us four and no more" was the way Yogananda described their attitude. America wasn't yet ready for world-brotherhood colonies.

But Master knew that, eventually, his dream must be fulfilled.

27

Attunement

ASTER WAS TO SPEAK one Sunday morning at Hollywood Church, when Sue and Bud Clewell, my relatives in Westwood Village, came to visit me. After the service, Master invited us to join him for lunch.

A small group of us ate on the stage behind the closed curtains. This afternoon was my first opportunity to observe Master in the role of host. It was a charming experience. His total lack of affectation, delightful wit, gentle courtesy, and warm, kindly laughter which included everyone in his joy, would have enchanted any audience.

Among those present were Dr. and Mrs. Lewis. A lady inquired, "Master, Dr. Lewis was your first disciple in this country, wasn't he?"

Master's response was unexpectedly reserved. "That's what they say," he replied quietly. His tone, even more than his words, made such a marked contrast to the affability he had been showing that the lady seemed quite taken aback. Noticing her surprise, Master explained more kindly, "I never speak of people as my disciples. God is the Guru: They are *His* disciples."

To Master, discipleship was too sacred a subject to be treated lightly, even in casual conversation.

Sue and Bud found Master charming. "But," Sue challenged me a little belligerently, later, "why do you call him 'Master'? This is a free country! Anyway, no one has a right to be master of another human being!"

"Sue, it isn't our freedom we've given him. It's our bondage! I've never known anyone so respectful of the freedoms of others. We call him 'Master' in the sense of teacher. He is a true master of the practices in which we ourselves are struggling to excel."

Sue's objection to our loving appellation for our guru was by no means unusual. Perhaps if a master were to appear on the stage of life like some Nietzschean Zarathustra, making grand pronouncements on obscure themes that no one in his right mind had ever thought of before, people, mistaking their bewilderment for awe, might cry, "Ah, here indeed is a *master*." But masters usually live more or less prosaically. They get born in mangers. They teach familiar truths in simple ways. One might say they almost flaunt their ordinariness. Human nature doesn't take kindly to greatness in mere *people*. And it is in their perfect humanity that masters most truly reveal their greatness.

People rarely see that the greatness of God's ways, as expressed through the lives of His awakened children, lies in a transcendent view of mundane realities, and not in a rigid denial of these realities. From the thought, "Nothing is divine," man must grow to the realization, "All things are divine."

Our "bondage" to Master was a "bondage" purely of love. He, far more than we, appreciated the sacredness of this relationship, and treated it with the deepest dignity and respect. But where love was missing on a disciple's part, the bond broke, or was never formed. And then even disciples were known to lose sight of what it meant to call their guru, "Master."

"I didn't come here," they complained, "to pour *cement!*" No? Why, then, did you come?

"Why, to meditate, of course, to attain *samadhi*."

And did you imagine that *samadhi* would come in any other way than by attunement with your guru?

"Well, no. After all that's why I came here. But what has attunement got to do with pouring cement? It's in my meditations that I need his help."

O blind ones, can't you see that self-transformation is a *total* process? that what the Master gives us spiritually must be perceived on *every* level of our existence? that no real difference exists between God in the form of cement and God in the form of blissful visions?

Rare, alas, is that disciple who feels no inner resistance, born of egotism, to complete acceptance of his guru. "I want to express my own creativity!" is a complaint frequently thought, less frequently expressed. O foolish devotee, don't you see that man has *nothing* to express that he can call truly his own? that his ideas, his opinions, his so-called "inspirations"—all, *all* but reflect currents of consciousness that are equally available to everyone? Only by attunement to God's will can we truly express *ourselves*.

For disciples, the surest way to express themselves creatively is to attune themselves to their guru's wishes. His entire task is to speed them on the path of self-unfoldment.

There were times when I myself felt that Master had erred in some matter, or had not sufficiently grasped some point. There was even a time, as you will see in a later chapter, when my questioning took the form of more serious doubts. But always I found, in time, that he was the one who was right. His actions, unusual though they sometimes were, were based on sure intuitions that, incredibly, always worked out for the best.

Had we listened more sensitively to the subtle nuances of his guidance, I almost think we could have changed the world. Certainly we would all have radically transformed ourselves.

Master had, albeit reluctantly, to abandon his dream of personally founding a world-brotherhood colony in Encinitas. Thereafter he turned his mind to organizing the existing communities along more strictly monastic lines. Several of the monks waxed critical that things hadn't been organized long before. New as I was in the work, I looked up to these men as my superiors on the path. It didn't occur to me that they were actually being negative.

Master's way was, if possible, to let the disciples play out their fantasies, that they might learn from them. I was never really brought fully into the present picture, but one day Boone, a fellow monk, came charging into my room to announce grandly, "Master has appointed a committee. He wants you and me to be on it."

"A committee? What does he want us to do?"

"We're to organize the work."

"What aspects of it?"

"All aspects of it—everything!" Boone swept an arm outward in an expansive gesture.

"Well," I said, dubiously, "if Master says so. But I don't really know much about the work. I can't imagine how he expects me to help organize it!"

"Oh, you won't have to do much. Just lend a hand whenever we ask for it."

It turned out I didn't really have to do anything. For some weeks various members of the committee met by twos and threes, informally, to discuss everything they felt needed changing. There was much talk, some complaining, and little action. Gradually, complaints assumed the dominant role. The main office, Boone informed me indignantly, was obstructing the committee's work, and thereby, of course, Master's will. I felt incompetent to offer positive suggestions, but shared my fellow members' indignation.

One day Boone dashed into my room in a burst of anger. "Miss Sahly completely refuses to obey the committee's latest directive!"

Why this was unthinkable! I rose to my feet. "We must go speak to her!" Together we strode over to the main office. I told Miss Sahly (now Shraddha Mata) that in refusing to cooperate with the committee she was disobeying Master, that the matter in question was a committee decision, and that, for the welfare of the work, she must absolutely accept it.

"You young hotheads!" Master cried when he learned about the episode. "What do you mean, bursting in there and shouting like that?" He proceeded to give me, in particular, the best tongue-lashing I ever heard him give anyone.

I was aghast. I had pictured myself bravely striking blows in his cause, only to find myself fighting on the wrong side! Miss Sahly, it turned out, was a highly respected disciple of many years' standing, and a member of the Board of Directors. Master, moreover, had never told her, nor anyone else, that our committee had any special powers.

Running out of things to say about our office invasion, but finding himself still in fine voice, Master started in on the committee itself. He called it "do-nothing, negative, a complete farce." Most of the monks, including the other committee members, were present. Master's entire tirade, however, was directed at me.

But Master, I thought, *I took hardly any part in the committee's activities!* Outwardly silent, I couldn't help feeling a little resentment at what I considered my undeserved humiliation. Later, I reflected that my reaction only proved all the more my need for criticism.

"Sir," I pleaded earnestly that evening, "please scold me more often."

"I understand." He looked at me keenly. "But what you need is more devotion."

It was true. In heeding the negative criticisms of my older brothers I had fallen—from what had seemed to me good motives—into judgmental attitudes, which are forever inimical to love.

Soon afterwards I approached Master. "I'm sorry, Sir," I said.

"That's the way!" Master smiled lovingly. From then on the incident was closed between us.

Master discouraged negativity even in a good cause. A couple of years later a certain man tried by trickery to hurt the work in one of our churches. Mr. Jacot, a loyal and devoted member, uncovered the man's schemes and denounced him publicly. Master expressed his gratitude to Mr. Jacot afterwards for saving us from a perilous situation. After thanking him, however, he gently scolded him for the means he had employed. "It is not good," he said, "regardless of one's intentions, to create wrong vibrations through anger and harsh words. The good that you have accomplished would have been greater had you employed peaceful means."

It was several days after the committee episode that I first met Daya Mata (then Faye Wright), now the president of SRF. I was in the main office after working-hours. A youthful-looking woman of radiant countenance entered the room. I sensed in her a deep attunement with Master. Seeing me, she paused, then addressed me pleasantly.

"You're Donald, aren't you? I'm Faye. I've heard about you." She smiled. "My, that was quite a stir you boys created with that committee of yours!"

I felt acutely embarrassed. As far as I was concerned, that committee was a dead issue. But she, not knowing how I stood on the matter, decided to help me to understand it better. As we conversed, I found myself thinking, "So this is an example of those disciples who were supposed to be 'obstructing' Master's wishes. I'd a thousand times rather be like her than like any of those complainers!" Her calm self-possession, kindliness, and transparent devotion to Master impressed me deeply. From now on, I resolved, I would look upon her as my model in the ideal spirit of discipleship that I was striving to acquire.

"We must learn to give up self-will if we want to please Master. And that," she added significantly, "is what we are trying to do."

Simple teaching, simply expressed! But it rang true. What, I thought, reflecting on her words, was the use of building this, of organizing that, of doing even the most laudable work, if *Master* was not pleased? For his job was to express God's will for each of us. To please him was, quite simply, to please God.

Let others do the important, outward things, I decided. For me only one thing would matter from now on: to do Master's will, *to please him.*

Ironically, it was very soon afterward—almost as if in response to my determination to court obscurity—that Master singled me out for responsibility. He put me in charge of the monks at Mt. Washington.

Several weeks passed. Then one day I was standing with Herbert Freed, one of the ministers, outside the entrance to the basement. We were talking with Master, who was on the point of going out for a drive. Herbert was to leave that afternoon to become the minister of our church in Phoenix, Arizona, and Master was giving him last-minute instructions. After a pause, Master continued quietly:

"You have a great work to do."

Turning to Herbert, I smiled my felicitations.

"It is you I'm talking to, Walter," Master corrected me. Moments later his car drove away. To what sort of work had he been referring?

Thereafter, he often repeated this prediction.

What was this "great work"? Master's words were, in their cumulative effect at least, the most insistent he ever addressed to me. They returned often to my mind, demanding comprehension. Clearly, I reflected, they had been meant as a command, not as a compliment. They seemed intended to invest me with a sense of personal responsibility for some aspect of his mission, and also, perhaps, to inspire me not to shirk that responsibility. Instinctively I feared such responsibility.

But when, one time, I resisted Master's efforts to draw me into teaching activities, his response was brusque. "Living for God," he said sternly, "is martyrdom!"

28

Reincarnation

ABOATLOAD OF FISHERMEN in Encinitas had had a bad day. After hours of work, and very little to show for it, they were ready to go home. Paramhansa Yogananda happened to be out strolling on the beach when they brought their boat in.

"You are giving up?" he inquired.

"No fish," they replied sadly.

"Why don't you try just once more?"

Something in his manner made them heed his advice. Going out once more, they got a large haul.

And thus was added another puzzling item to a growing legend in the local community of Encinitas about the strange, kindly Swami around whom things seemed somehow always to happen for the best.

To me this story, which I heard indirectly from some of the townsfolk there, illustrates a basic truth of human life, one that Master often emphasized: No matter how many times a person fails, he should never accept failure as the final judgment of Destiny. As children of the Infinite, we have a right to God's infinite bounty. Failure is *never* His will for us. It is merely a temporary condition that we impose on ourselves through some flaw in our attunement with cosmic law. By repeated efforts to succeed, we gradually refine that attunement. "Try just once more," Master said. If our intentions are lawful, failure simply means we haven't yet succeeded. Life, in other words, gives us our failures as stepping stones to success.

The story of the fishermen also suggests that God's forgiveness— call it, rather, His loving expectation of us—is eternal. The teachings of India claim that we have an eternity of opportunities to achieve perfection. We ought never to abandon hope, even if failure dogs us all our life. Through repeated incarnations we *must* succeed, eventually.

On the subject of reincarnation, Indian philosophy seems at odds with Christian teachings. But in fact this doctrine is denied only in the prevailing *interpretations* of the Bible, and not in the Bible itself. Reincarnation is not an *un-Christian* teaching. Nor, for that matter, is it an un-Jewish one. It was taught by some of the great early Christian Fathers, including Origen (A.D. 185-254),* who claimed to have received it in an unbroken tradition "from apostolic times." Indeed, it was not until five centuries after Christ, in 553 A.D., at the Second Council of Constantinople, that this doctrine was finally removed from Christian dogma. The anathema that was pronounced against it was a consequence of political maneuverings, not of theological purism. Scholars have discovered that Pope Vigilius, although present in Constantinople at that time, took no part in pronouncing the anathema, and in fact boycotted the Council altogether.

Numerous Biblical passages† support belief in reincarnation. This

---

*The Encyclopedia Britannica calls Origen "The most prominent of all the Church Fathers with the possible exception of Augustine." Origen wrote, of reincarnation, "Is it not reasonable that souls should be introduced into bodies in accordance with their merits and previous deeds?"

†"But thou, Bethlehem Ephratah, though thou be little among the thousands of

doctrine may be found, subsequent to Biblical times, in Jewish as well as in Christian traditions. Rabbi Manasseh ben Israel (1604-1657 A.D.), Jewish theologian and statesman, wrote, "The belief or the doctrine of the transmigration of souls is a firm and infallible dogma accepted by the whole assemblage of our church [*sic*] with one accord, so that there is none to be found who dare to deny it. . . . The truth of it has been incontestably demonstrated by the Zohar, and all the books of the Kabalists." And while modern Jews generally reject this doctrine, rabbis familiar with the spiritual traditions of Judaism do not endorse their rejection. Reincarnation is endorsed in the *Shulhan Oruch*, which is the major book of laws in the *Torah*. A student for the Rabbinate in Israel has sent me several supportive quotations from this book, including these words from the *Sha'ar Hatsiyune*, letter 6vav: "That soul will be sent time and time again to this world until he does what God wants him to do." The student said that his Rabbi, after reading this letter, could no longer deny the doctrine of reincarnation.

Judah, yet out of thee shall he come forth unto me that is to be ruler in Israel; whose goings forth have been from old, from everlasting." (Micah 5:2.)

"For all the prophets and the law prophesied until John. And if ye will receive it, this is Elias, which was for to come. He that hath ears to hear, let him hear." (Matthew 11:13-15.)

"And as they came down from the mountain, Jesus charged them, saying, Tell the vision [of his transfiguration, in which he had revealed himself as the Messiah] to no man, until the Son of Man be risen again from the dead. And his disciples asked him, saying, Why then say the scribes that Elias must first come? And Jesus answered and said unto them, Elias truly shall first come, and restore all things. But I say unto you, That Elias is come already, and they knew him not, but have done unto him whatsoever they listed. Likewise shall also the Son of Man suffer of them. Then the disciples understood that he spake unto them of John the Baptist." (Matthew 17:9-13.)

"Him that overcometh will I make a pillar in the temple of my God, *and he shall go no more out.*" (Revelation 3:12.)

The above passages present a small selection, merely, out of many in the Bible that demonstrate support for the doctrine of reincarnation. Christian traditionalists would be wise to question some of the *sources* for their own traditions. Do those sources derive from great saints, who knew God? Or are they merely deductions founded on reason, not on actual spiritual experience?

Among famous Westerners who have subscribed to this doctrine, the German philosopher Schopenhauer wrote: "Were an Asiatic to ask me for a definition of Europe, I should be forced to answer him: It is that part of the world which is haunted by the incredible delusion that man was created out of nothing, and that his present birth is his first entrance into life."* Voltaire wrote, "It is not more surprising to be born twice than once." And the British philosopher Hume stated that reincarnation is "the only system to which Philosophy can hearken."

According to this doctrine, life on earth is a school containing many grades. Our ultimate goal is graduation from limited, egoic awareness into cosmic consciousness. Stepping stones to this unconditioned awareness are the removal of all confining attachments and desires, the expansion of love, and a growing realization that God is the one underlying Reality of the universe.

The results of self-effort are regulated by the law of karma. (Newton's law of action and reaction is a material manifestation of this spiritual law.) According to karmic law, every action, even of thought, engenders its own balancing reaction. Hatred given results in hatred received. Love given attracts love. Karma may be described as the system of rewards and punishments by which the ego learns ultimately to manifest its innate divine nature. Suffering is the karmic result of action that, in some way, is out of tune with that true nature. Fulfillment is the reward for living, to some degree at least, in harmony with that nature.

People often object, "If everyone reincarnates, why is it that no one remembers having lived before?" The simple answer is that many do remember!

One of the most interesting accounts of this nature ever to come to my attention was sent to me years ago by a friend in Cuba, where it had been reprinted in the newspapers from an article that appeared first in France. According to the account, a young French girl, the child of devout Catholic parents, had been using recognizably Indian words, such as "rupee," as soon as she was old enough to speak. Two words that she used repeatedly were, "Wardha," and "Bapu." Her parents, intrigued, began reading books on India. Wardha, they

---

Parerga and Paralipomena.

learned, was the village where Mahatma Gandhi had established his ashram. And "Bapu" was the familiar nickname by which intimate friends and disciples knew him. The child claimed that in her last life she had lived in Wardha with Bapu.

One day someone presented her parents with a copy of *Autobiography of a Yogi,* in the latter part of which Yogananda describes his visit, in 1936, to Mahatma Gandhi in Wardha. The moment the child saw Yogananda's photograph on the jacket, she cried gleefully, "Oh, that's Yogananda! He came to Wardha. He was very beautiful!"

Belief in the principle of rebirth helps one to view progress joyously, without fear and self-doubt.

"Is there any end to evolution?" a visitor once asked Paramhansa Yogananda.

"No end," the Master replied. "Progress goes on until you achieve endlessness."

At Mt. Washington we took it quite in stride if ever Master told us, as he sometimes did, about our own or someone else's past lives.

I once told him I had always wanted to live alone. His reply was, "That is because you have done it before. Most of those who are with me have lived alone many times in the past." He made such remarks so casually that it rarely occurred to me to ask him for more information.

A few years after Dr. Lewis lost his mother, Master, knowing Doctor's devotion to her, informed him, "She has been reborn. If you go to . . ." he mentioned some address in New England, "you will find her there." Dr. Lewis made the journey.

"It was uncanny," he told me. "The child was only three years old, but in many of her mannerisms she seemed exactly like my mother. I observed, too, that she took an instantaneous liking to me."

Discussions on reincarnation sometimes became intensely interesting. One day I asked Master, "Did Judas have any spiritual realization?"

"He had some bad karma, of course," Master replied, "but all the same, he was a prophet."

"He *was?*"

"Oh, yes," Master asserted emphatically. "He had to be, to be one of the twelve. But he had to go through two thousand years of suffering for his treachery. He was liberated finally in this century, in India. Jesus appeared to a certain master there and asked him to free him. I knew Judas in this life," Master added.

"You did! What was he like?"

"Always very quiet and by himself. He still had a little attachment to money. One day another disciple began poking fun at him for this tendency. But the master shook his head. 'Don't,' he said quietly. 'Leave him alone.' "

Sometimes Master intrigued us with references, always casual, to the past lives of certain well-known public figures. "Winston Churchill," he told us, "was Napoleon. Napoleon wanted to conquer England. Churchill, as England's Prime Minister, has fulfilled that ambition. Napoleon wanted to destroy England. As Churchill he has had to preside over the disintegration of the British Empire. Napoleon was sent into exile, then returned again to power. Churchill, similarly, was sent out of politics, then after some time came back to power again."

It is an interesting fact that Churchill, as a young man, found inspiration in the military exploits of Napoleon.

"Hitler," Master continued, "was Alexander the Great." An interesting point of comparison here is that, in warfare, both Hitler and Alexander employed the strategy of lightening attack—*blitzkrieg,* as Hitler called it. In the Orient, of course, where Alexander's conquests were responsible for the destruction of great civilizations, his appellation, "the Great," is quoted sarcastically.

Master had hoped to reawaken in Hitler Alexander's well-known interest in the teachings of India, and thereby to steer the dictator's ambitions toward more spiritual goals. He actually attempted to see Hitler in 1935, but his request for an interview was denied.

Mussolini, Master said, was Marc Anthony. Kaiser Wilhelm was Julius Caesar. Stalin was Genghis Khan.

"Who was Franklin Roosevelt?" I inquired.

"I've never told anybody," Master replied with a wry smile. "I was afraid I'd get into trouble!"

Master knew the value of offsetting abstract teachings with these interesting sidelights on reality. The barriers to memory raised between lifetimes to the average person melt away before the man of wisdom. But of course Master's real interest, and ours, lay in our attainment of divine enlightenment. We found that familiarity with the law of reincarnation helped us to deepen our determination to escape the monotonous round of death and rebirth.

Human life, the Scriptures of India tell us, is a dream. Its ultimate goal is to help us to learn well our lessons, to overcome our attachments to material limitations, and to realize that all things, seemingly real in themselves, are but manifestations of the one light of God. The highest lesson of all is to learn to love God. The best karma of all is the ability to love Him.

"Sir," Norman once said, rather morosely, to Master, "I don't believe I have very good karma."

"Remember this," Master replied with deep earnestness, "it takes very, *very*, VERY good karma even to *want* to know God!"

Through love of God, and only through that love, may one win final release from physical rebirth, and the right to advance to higher spheres of existence. Victory comes not by hating this world, but by beholding God's presence in it everywhere, by paying reverence to the veriest fool as though before a holy shrine.

"You must be very joyous and happy," Master said, "because this is God's dream, and the little man and the big man are all nothing but the Dreamer's consciousness."

29

Gardens—
Mundane And Spiritual

SOMETIME DURING AUGUST or September, 1949, Paramhansa Yogananda acquired his last and most beautiful ashram property: twelve acres shaped by Nature into a steep-sided bowl surrounding a miniature lake. This "Lake Shrine," as Master named it, nestles serenely in the arms of a broad curve formed by Sunset Boulevard as, leaving the town of Pacific Palisades, it makes its final sweep down to the ocean. The property is one of the loveliest I have seen in a lifetime of world travel.

Soon after Master obtained this property, he invited the monks out to see it. Walking its grounds, we were wonderstruck at their beauty. Happily Master predicted, "This will be a showcase for the work!" Later on he had us don bathing suits and enter the water with him.

"I am sending the divine light all through this lake," he said. "This is holy water now. Whoever comes here in future will receive a divine blessing."

Even today, nearly thirty years after that event, merely to enter those grounds is to feel their spiritual power.

Soon we began the task of preparing it for a public opening one year later. Trees, shrubs, and flowers were planted on the steep hillsides. Statues of leading figures in the great world religions were placed picturesquely about the grounds, to emphasize the basic oneness of all religions. ("Where do you want the Buddha to sit?" we inquired one day. Master was standing nearby. "The Buddha," he replied with a quiet smile, "prefers to remain standing.")

In the early months of preparation, swarms of gnats proved an extreme nuisance. The fascination they demonstrated for our eyes, ears, and nostrils was anything but flattering. "Master," I exclaimed in exasperation one day, "what irony! Why must this beautiful setting be spoiled by these flies?"

Calmly Master replied, "That is the Lord's way of keeping us ever moving toward Him."

Happily, the Lord found other ways to accomplish this objective. The gnats proved only a temporary pest.

One day we were moving a delicate but rather heavy tropical plant into position on the hillside. Our handling evidently was too rough, for Master cried out, "Be careful! Can't you *feel?* It's alive!"

His sensitivity to all things living inspired sensitivity from them in return. Even plants seemed to respond. His gardens flourished. Tropical mangoes and bananas grew at Mt. Washington, where the climate is not conducive to their survival. Shraddha Mata (Miss Sahly) tells of one day watching what she calls a "rose devotee" that kept turning in its vase to face Master as he moved about the room. "Plants," Master explained, "have a degree of consciousness." Above all, like every sentient being, they respond to love.

Sometimes in his training he likened us, too, to plants. Of a monk who had been resisting his counsel, he exclaimed, "What a job one takes on when he tries to improve people! He has to go into their minds and see what it is they are thinking. The rose in the vase looks beautiful; one forgets all the care that went into growing it. But if it takes such care to produce a rose, how much more care is needed to develop a perfect human being!"

Like a divine gardener, Master labored unceasingly for our spiritual development. It took patience, love, courage, and considerably greater faith in us than most of us had in ourselves. For where we saw only our own egos struggling to shed their imperfections, he saw our souls struggling to reclaim their divine birthright in God. Some of his disciples justified his faith in them better than others did, but he extended to all the same vision of their ultimate perfectibility.

At Twenty-Nine Palms in October, 1949, Master said to me, "Those who are with me"—he must have meant, *in tune with me*—"I never have any trouble with. Just a glance with the eyes is enough. It is much better when I can teach that way." He added, "They are saints from before, most of them."

Another time he told me, "Many of the disciples will find freedom in this life."

Of the disciples, the one who was the most generous with his anecdotes about Master was Dr. Lewis, the first Kriya Yogi in America, and by now highly advanced on the spiritual path. We would sit for hours with Doctor while he regaled us with stories, some of them amusing, some serious, all of them instructive. They helped us to see how the relationship between guru and disciple evolves gradually into one of divine friendship in God.

Towad the end of October of that year Dr. Lewis and several others accompanied Master to San Francisco to meet India's Prime Minister, Jawaharlal Nehru. Doctor returned to Mt. Washington with tales of their journey, then went on to share with us other reminiscences of his years of association with Master.

Master and his little group had visited a Chinese restaurant in San Francisco. The "vegetarian" meal they'd requested had been served with bits of chicken in it. A lady in the group, a prominent member of another religious organization, had stormed angrily into the kitchen and denounced the staff for this "outrage."

"Master," Doctor told us, "considered an uncontrolled temper a 'sin' far worse than the relatively minor one of eating chicken. 'It's not important enough to make a fuss over,' he remarked to the rest of us. Pushing the bits of meat to one side, he calmly ate the rest of his meal."

That night Master and the Lewises had adjoining hotel rooms. "Master kept the door open between us," Doctor said. "I knew he didn't really want us to sleep that night. He himself never sleeps, you know. Not, at least, the way you and I do; he's always in superconsciousness. And he wants to break *us*, too, of too much dependence on subconsciousness—'counterfeit *samadhi*,' he calls it.

So I guess he saw here an opportunity for us to spend a few hours sharing spiritual friendship and inspiration with him. We don't get many chances for that any more, now that the work has become worldwide.

"The problem was, Mrs. Lewis and I were both tired—she especially so. We'd been traveling all day. 'We're going to sleep,' she announced in a tone of finality. That, as far as she was concerned, was that.

"But Master had other ideas.

"Mrs. Lewis and I went to bed. Master, with apparent submissiveness, lay down on his bed. I was just getting relaxed, and Mrs. Lewis was beginning to drift peacefully off to sleep, when suddenly Master, as though with infinite relevance, said:

" 'Sub gum.'

"Nothing more. Sub gum was the name of one of those Chinese dishes we'd eaten earlier that day. I smiled to myself. But Mrs. Lewis muttered grimly, 'He's *not* going to make me get up!' A few minutes passed. We were just drifting off again. Suddenly, in marveling tones:

" 'Sub gum *duff!*' Master pronounced the words carefully, like a child playing with unaccustomed sounds.

"Desperately Mrs. Lewis whispered, 'We're sleeping!' She turned for help to the wall.

"More minutes passed. Then, very slowly:

" '*Super* sub gum duff!' The words this time were spoken earnestly, like a child in the process of making some important discovery.

"By this time I was chuckling to myself. But though sleep was beginning to seem to both of us rather an 'impossible dream,' Mrs. Lewis was still hanging on fervently to her resolution.

"More minutes passed. And then the great discovery:

" 'Super SUBMARINE sub gum duff!' "

"Further resistance was impossible! Howling with merriment, we rose from the bed. For the remainder of the night sleep was forgotten. We talked and laughed with Master. Gradually the conversation shifted to serious matters. We ended up speaking only of God, then meditating. With his blessings we felt no further need for sleep that night.

Dr. Lewis, finding us keenly receptive to his good humor this evening, related another anecdote. "Master and I were standing on a sidewalk one day many years ago," he said, "when a man riding by on his bicycle noticed Master's long hair, and stuck his tongue out at him derisively. About two feet further on he came to a large mud puddle. Right in the middle of that puddle the front wheel of his bicycle came off. He went sprawling!"

Gradually, Doctor's reminiscences grew more serious. They took him back to his early days with Master.

"There was a man who'd been condemned to death for a crime that many felt he hadn't committed. The day before his scheduled execution I was with Master, and mentioned this case to him. Master became very pensive. Silently he retired to a corner of the room, and sat there quietly. After some time he returned to our circle with a smile, and resumed conversation. He never mentioned the condemned man. The following morning, however, the news came out in the papers: At the eleventh hour, the governor had issued a pardon.

"You know, we weren't as familiar in those days with Master's methods as you all are now. We didn't know the wonderful things he could do. For that matter, we didn't know what *any* master can do. By now, people have had years to get to know him better. It was more difficult then for us to have the kind of faith you all have in him. In that episode of the condemned man, for instance, Master never told us he'd done anything to help him. He rarely speaks of the wonderful things he does. It's just that, when things keep on happening around him, you begin to wonder. On that occasion, it was only after the reprieve that I began to suspect strongly that Master had had a hand in the matter.

"You see, he doesn't want to amaze us with miracles. Love is the force by which he seeks to draw us to God."

As we left Dr. Lewis late that evening, we thanked him from our hearts for so generously sharing with us his unique experiences.

At about this time in my life Master began asking me to jot down his words, intimating that he wanted me someday to write about him. For hours he would reminisce with me about his life, his experiences in establishing the work, his hopes and plans for its future. He told me countless stories, some to illustrate points he was making; others, I suppose, simply because they were interesting, or helped in some general way to round out my understanding of the path. Many of his meanings reached me not only through the medium of words and stories, but by a kind of osmosis, a subtle impression gathered from a facial expression, or from the tone of his voice, or by some even subtler transferral of consciousness.

One day I asked him, "What are the most important qualities on the spiritual path?"`

"Deep sincerity," Master replied, "and devotion. It isn't the number of years one spends on the path that counts, but how deeply one tries to find God. Jesus said, 'The first shall be last, and the last, first.'

"I once met a lady in the state of Washington. She was eighty years old, and all her life she'd been an atheist. By God's grace, at our meeting she became converted to this path. Thereafter she sought God intensely. For the better part of every day, whenever she wasn't meditating, she would play a recording of my poem, 'God! God! God!' She lived only a few years longer, but in that short time she attained liberation."

On Christmas Day that year we enjoyed our traditional banquet. Before the banquet, place cards had been set out on the tables; the affair had been planned as a restricted family gathering. But at the last moment, numbers of guests had arrived uninvited. Room was courteously made for them, some of the renunciates offering their own seats.

In the office afterwards, a few of us were discussing with Master the inconvenience that had been caused by the sudden influx of people. A monk expressed his distress at their presumption. But I had been fortunate to observe another aspect of the episode.

"Sir," I said, "the disciples were vying with one another for the privilege of giving up their seats."

"Ah!" Master smiled blissfully. "Those are the things that please me!"

30

A Divine Test

FOR SOME TIME after the Christmas holidays, my meditations were blissful. But after a month or so, subtle delusions began to enter my mind. First came pride, in the feeling that this joy separated me from others—not, I believe, in the sense of making me think myself better than they, but in the equally false sense of holding me aloof from outward interests, however innocent. This state of consciousness masqueraded as wisdom, but in fact was born of my spiritual inexperience. For the devotee should learn to see God outside himself as well as inside—outside especially in wholesome activities and in beautiful things. The world we live in is, after all, God's world. To reject it is, in a sense, to reject Him. Pride follows such rejection, and with pride, the temptation to take personal credit for whatever inspirations one feels.

From pride there developed increasing tension in my spiritual efforts. And then, realizing that I needed to become more humble, I *grasped* at inner guidance, as I had been grasping at joy. I fell a prey to what the Roman Catholics call "scrupulosity."

At about this time, Master went to Twenty-Nine Palms to complete his commentary on the *Bhagavad Gita*. He took me with him. Weeks in Master's company would, I hoped, banish the turmoil that had been building up within me.

It was wonderful to listen to him as he worked on his writings. He would simply look up into the Spiritual Eye, then speak with hardly a pause, while his secretary raced to keep up with him on the typewriter.

I got to spend several days at Master's place. But after that he instructed me to stay at the monks' retreat and go through the old SRF magazines, clipping out his *Gita* commentaries and "editing" them.

Editing? I knew this particular assignment had already been given to another, senior disciple.

I'd gone to the desert with high hopes of spending every day with him. It was particularly distressing now to find myself completely alone. Unaccustomed to solitude, I felt abandoned utterly. Intense moods began to assail me.

I felt as though two forces were opposing each other within me. Bravely I tried to give strength to the good side by meditating hours daily, but the very effort of meditation only deepened my sense of hopelessness.

Master once told an audience, "I used to think Satan was only a human invention, but now I know, and add my testimony to that of others who lived before me, that Satan is a reality. He is a universal, conscious force whose sole aim is to keep all beings bound to the wheel of delusion." What I felt now was that God and Satan, warring inside me, were beating *me* up in their efforts to get at one another! It was not that I had the slightest wish to return to a worldly life. That desire, with God's grace, has never for a moment entered my heart since I first set foot on the spiritual path. What was happening, rather, was that, while I longed for inner peace, I found myself unaccountably terrified of going deep in meditation, where alone true peace can be found.

The worst of my ordeal, however, was that while it lasted I wasn't even able to call on Master with my accustomed faith. Suddenly I found myself plunged into violent doubts. It was not that I doubted his goodness, or his spiritual greatness, or even my commitment to him as my guru. But the thought suddenly forced itself upon me insidiously: "He lacks wisdom." It was an idea over which I had no control. There was no question of my *entertaining* these doubts. I would have done anything to be rid of them; they made me utterly miserable.

My doubt illustrates more or less typically the problem of every devotee. Before he can attain divine freedom, he must weed out every obstructing tendency that he has carried over from the past. Mere intellectual affirmation of victory is not enough: He must also face his delusions in stern hand-to-hand combat. Each seeker has his own special, self-created delusions to overcome. But overcome them he must, if he is to advance on the path.

"You are doubting now," Master told me one day, "because you doubted in the past."

During this inner test, it was never that Master was indifferent to my welfare. Rather he tried in various ways to reassure me. But it was his way never to intrude on our free will to the point where it would mean fighting our important battles for us. That would have deprived us of the opportunity to develop our own strength.

I was touched by his anxiety to comfort me. But for me, the important result of this test was that I knew now, more deeply than ever before, that I belonged to him, and that the outward ups and downs of the path didn't really matter so long as I felt his love in my heart.

31

The "Bhagavad Gita"

"A NEW SCRIPTURE HAS BEEN BORN!" Master spoke ecstatically. His commentary on the *Bhagavad Gita* had been finished. In three months of unbroken dictation he had completed 1,500 pages.

Master and I were walking around the compound of his retreat. Having finished his manuscript, he had summoned me at last to help him with suggestions for the preliminary editing.

"A new Scripture has been born!" he repeated. "Millions will find God through this book. Not just thousands. Millions! I *know*. I have seen it."

My first task, now that I'd been brought out of seclusion, was to read the entire manuscript through and get an over-all feeling for it. I found the experience almost overwhelming. Never before had I read anything so deep, and at the same time so beautiful and uplifting. To think that only recently I had been questioning Master's wisdom! I kicked myself mentally for being such a chump. His book was filled with the deepest wisdom I had ever encountered. Unlike most philosophical works, moreover, it was fresh and alive, each page a sparkling rill of original insights. With the sure touch of a master teacher, profound truths were lightened occasionally with graceful humor, or with charming and instructive stories, or highlighted with brief touches of new, sometimes startling information, and constantly clarified, as Master himself said exultingly, with "illustration after illustration."

"I understand now," he told me, "why my master never let me read other *Gita* interpretations. Had I done so, my mind might have been influenced by the opinions they expressed. But this book came entirely from God. It is not philosophy—the mere *love* of wisdom: It *is* wisdom. To make sure I didn't write it from a level of opinion, I tuned in with Byasa's* consciousness before beginning my dictation. Everything I said was what he himself intended."

My three months of seclusion were over; there now followed two months of concentrated work with Master at his place. I spent many hours in his company.

It puzzled me at first why Master would want anyone to edit his writings for him. They were so manifestly inspired, and—well, I thought, didn't divine inspiration imply perfection on *every* level? Not necessarily, it seemed. Inspiration, Master explained, lies primarily in the vibrations and the ideas expressed.

Logical sentence structure, I gradually realized, like good plumbing, belongs to this physical plane of existence. It is a tool merely, of thought and communication. Cerebration is slow and ponderous compared to the soul's transcendent intuitions. Many times it has happened that an important scientific discovery appeared full blown in the mind of its discoverer, only to require years of plodding work for him to present that intuitive insight clearly and convincingly to others.

As Master once said to me, "By helping me with editing, you

---

*The ancient author of the *Bhagavad Gita.*

yourself evolve." Master could cope easily and efficiently with mundane problems, including those of grammar and literary style, when he had a mind to. As he once told me, "I did edit one book myself: *Whispers from Eternity*." And this I considered not only one of his finest works, but one of the loveliest books of poetry ever written.* In editing his *Gita* commentaries, however, Master invited our suggestions, and seemed content to pursue much of his work on the basis of them.

Other monks came out on weekends, and sometimes for longer visits. To a group of us one day Master told of an amusing occurrence during his months of dictation. Jerry had taken a notion to cover the roof of Master's house with concrete. Over Master's objections, he insisted that such a roof would endure forever. "I then told him to finish the job right away," Master continued, "but Jerry said, 'It will be all right. I know what I am doing.' " Master was laughing. "First he put tar paper down on the roof. Then he nailed chicken wire over it. At this point the roof was a complete sieve: Hundreds of nails were sticking through it. 'Hurry up!' I urged. But Jerry saw no reason to rush things.

"Well, a huge storm came! Pans were put out frantically in every room. Water was dripping everywhere. The house was like a shower bath!

"But there were two rooms in which no water fell: the dictation room, and my bedroom. The roof was as much a sieve over these two as over the rest of the house, but Divine Mother didn't want my work to be interrupted. Only at the very end of the storm one drop fell into a bucket in the dictation room, and another one onto my bare stomach in the bedroom, while I lay relaxing on the bed. That was Divine Mother's way of playing a little joke on me!"

Jerry, who was present, said, "I'm sorry I'm so stubborn, Sir."

"Well, that's all right," Master spoke consolingly. "I attract stubborn people!"

One weekend Mrs. Harriet Grove, the leader of our center in Gardena, California, came out uninvited.

"This is the afternoon," Master told her, "that I usually go out for a ride in the car. But I knew you were coming, so I stayed home."

---

*I am referring to the 1929 and 1949 editions.

In the evenings, Master exercised by walking slowly around his retreat compound. Generally he asked me to accompany him. He was so much withdrawn from body-consciousness on those occasions that he sometimes had to lean on my arm for support. He would pause and sway back and forth, as if about to fall.

"I am in so many bodies," he remarked once, returning slowly to body-consciousness, "it is difficult for me to remember which body I am supposed to keep moving."

One day I was sitting in Master's dictation room, waiting while he worked on his *Gita* manuscript. While he wrote, his mind gravely focused on the task at hand, I gazed at him. How wonderful it was, I thought, to be his disciple. When he finished his work, he asked me to help him to his feet. Rising, he held my hands for a moment and gazed with joy into my eyes.

"Just a bulge of the ocean!" he said, softly.

In his *Gita* commentaries he had compared God to the ocean, and individual souls to its innumerable waves. "God is the Sole Reality manifesting through all beings," he said. I could see from his loving remark that he wanted my love to expand to embrace the Ocean of Spirit, of which his body was but a tiny expression.

32

"I Am Spirit"

ONE DAY at Twenty-Nine Palms, while Master was revising his *Bhagavad Gita* commentaries, he had sections of it read to a group of monks from Mt. Washington. The reading described the state of oneness with God. Once, Master had said, the devotee attains this divine state, he realizes that the Ocean of Spirit alone is real; God took on the appearance of his little ego; then, after a time, withdrew that wave into Himself again. In effect, the dream-child wakes up in cosmic consciousness to find himself God once more.

However, Master went on to explain, the saint who attains that exalted consciousness never says, "I am God," for he sees it was the vast Ocean that became his little wave of ego. The wave, in other words, would not claim, when referring to the little self, to be the Ocean.

Liberation from ego does not come with the first glimpses of cosmic consciousness. Present, at first, even in an expanded state of awareness, is the subtle memory, "I, the formless but nevertheless still real John Smith, am enjoying this state of consciousness." The body in this trance state is immobile; one's absorption in God at this point is called *sabikalpa samadhi*: qualified absorption, a condition that is still subject to change, for from it one returns to assume once again the limitations of ego. By repeated absorption in the trance state, however, ego's hold on the mind is gradually broken, until the realization dawns: "There is no John Smith to go back to. I am Spirit!" This is the supreme state: *nirbikalpa samadhi*, or unqualified absorption—a condition changeless and eternal. If from this state one returns to body-consciousness, it is no longer with the thought of separate existence from the ocean of Spirit. John Smith no longer exists: It is the eternal Spirit, now, which animates his body, eats through it, teaches through it, and carries on all the normal functions of a human being. This outward direction of energy on the part of one who has attained *nirbikalpa samadhi* is sometimes known also as *sahaja*, or effortless, *samadhi*.

Divine freedom comes only with the attainment of *nirbikalpa samadhi*. Until that stage the ego can still—and alas, sometimes does—draw the mind back down into delusion. With *nirbikalpa samadhi*, one becomes what is known as a *jivan mukta*, free even though living in a physical form. A *jivan mukta*, however, unimaginably high though his state is, is not yet *fully* emancipated. The subtle memory, "I am John Smith," has been destroyed; he can acquire no new karma, since the post of ego to which karma is tied has been broken. But there remains even now the memory of all those prior existences: John Smith in thousands, perhaps millions of incarnations; John Smith the one-time bandit, John Smith the disappointed musician, John Smith the betrayed lover, the beggar, the swaggering tyrant. All those old selves must be made over, their karma spiritualized, released into the Infinite.

"Very few saints on this earth have achieved final liberation," Master told me.

"Sir, why can't a master dissolve all his karma the moment he attains oneness with God?"

"Well," Master replied, "in that state you don't really care whether you come back or not. It is just like a dream to you then. You are awake, merely watching the dream. You can go on for incarnations that way, or you can say, 'I am free,' and *be* free right away. It's all in the mind. As soon as you say you are free, then you're free."

Referring to that degree of mental freedom which is a prior condition for even a glimpse of *samadhi*, he said, "It is only the thought that we are not free that keeps us from actually being free. Merely to break that thought would suffice to put us into *samadhi!* *Samadhi* is not something we have to *acquire*. We have it already!" Master added, "Dwell always on this thought: Eternally we have been with God. For a short time—for the fleeting breaths of a few incarnations—we are in delusion. Then again we are free in Him forever!"

When the soul attains final liberation, it becomes a *siddha* ("perfected being"), or *param mukta* ("supremely free soul"). Even in this state, individuality is not lost, but is retained in the form of memory. The karma of John Smith's many incarnations has been released into the Infinite, but the *memory* of them, now spiritualized, remains a fact throughout eternity. The soul, however, once it achieves this state of supreme liberation, rarely reactivates its own remembered individuality, and *never* does so except at the command of the Divine Will. When such a supremely free soul returns to this world, it comes only for the welfare of humanity. Such an incarnation is called an *avatar*, or "divine incarnation."

Such, Master told us, was Babaji, the first of our direct line of gurus. Such also were Lahiri Mahasaya—*yogavatar*, Master called him, or "incarnation of yoga"—and Swami Sri Yukteswar, whom Master identified as India's present-day *gyanavatar*, or "incarnation of wisdom."

"Sir," I asked Master one day at his desert retreat, "are *you* an *avatar?*"

With quiet simplicity he replied, "A work of this importance would have to be started by such a one."

An *avatar*, he told us, comes on earth with a divine mission, often for the general upliftment of mankind. The *siddha's* effort, by contrast, has necessarily been to unite his own consciousness perfectly with God's. God, therefore, does not work through *siddhas* in the same way that He works through *avatars*. To *avatars* He gives the power to bring vast numbers of souls to freedom in Him. To *siddhas* He gives the power to liberate themselves and a few others.

Though every great master is fully qualified to say, with Jesus, "I and my Father are one," many descend occasionally from that absolute state, as Jesus also did, to enjoy a loving "I-and-Thou" relationship with the Lord. The Indian Scriptures state that God created the universe "in order that He might enjoy Himself through many." The vast majority of His creatures, alas, have lost conscious touch with the infinite joy of their own being. The saints alone, in their joyous romance with the Lord, fulfill this deep and abiding purpose of His creation, by letting Him express His joy outwardly through their lives.

Avatars and other masters will often go through years of *sadhana* ("spiritual practice") in their youth, as an example to others. If they didn't, their disciples might claim that meditation and self-effort are not necessary for God-attainment, or perhaps simply that such practices are not their "way."

"If you want God," Master used to say, "go after Him. It takes great determination and steadfast, deep effort. And remember, the minutes are more important than the years."

33

"Original Christianity"

HOW DOES THE CONCEPT of *samadhi* agree with Christian teachings? Most church-goers, certainly, get no hint on Sunday mornings that the Bible promises them anything like cosmic consciousness. No one, however, has a "corner" on Christ's teachings, or for that matter on any religion.

Truth, like a diamond, is many-faceted. The teachings of Moses and Jesus Christ have been given certain emphases in the West, but other perfectly legitimate emphases are possible, and would reflect truths that have been cherished for centuries elsewhere in the world. Exposure to those unfamiliar traditions might prove enormously beneficial to Westerners who desire deeper insight into their own religious teachings.

It need surprise no one that the Bible means different things to different people. For is it not obvious that it cannot hold authority *beyond a person's own ability to understand it?* Jesus said, "Therefore I speak to them in parables: because they seeing see not; and hearing they hear not, neither do they understand." (Matthew 13:13.) Even after *explaining* his parable of the sower, he said, "Who hath ears to hear, let him hear." (Matthew 13:43.)

And what is it that determines one's ability to understand? Far more important than native intelligence is his actual, inner experience of divine truths. How else are they to be recognized?

As St. Anselm put it: "Who does not experience will not know. For just as experiencing a thing far exceeds the mere hearing of it, so the knowledge of him who experiences is beyond the knowledge of him who hears."

To return, then, to the question of Christian corroboration of the concept of *samadhi,* it is to the saints that we look first.

"The soul, when purified," wrote St. Catherine of Genoa, "abides entirely in God; its being is God."

St. Catherine of Sienna stated that Christ had told her in a vision, "I am That I am; thou art that which is not." In other words, the little vortex of her ego had no abiding reality of its own.

St. Veronica Giuliani, the Seventeenth-Century Capuchin nun, concerning her experience of mystical union, wrote in her *Diary* that she had received a conviction, far deeper than any intellectual concept or belief, that *"outside God nothing has any existence at all."*

St. Anselm wrote, "Not all of that joy shall enter into those who rejoice; but they who rejoice shall wholly enter into that joy."

Do not these quotations suggest persuasively that state which is known to Indian yogis as *samadhi?*

Let us see what Christian saints have said further on the subject of *infinity* as a definition of divine awareness.

"I, *who am infinite,*" wrote St. Catherine of Sienna, "seek infinite works—that is, an infinite perfection of love."

St. Bernard wrote, "Just as a little drop of water mixed with a lot of wine seems entirely to lose its own identity, while it takes on the taste of wine and its color . . . so it will inevitably happen that in saints every human affection will then, in some ineffable manner, melt away from self and be entirely transfused into the will of God."

"Is it not written in your law, I said, Ye are gods?" (John 10:34.) Thus Jesus answered the Jews, when they accused him of blasphemy for saying, "I and my Father are one."

"Thou art *That,*" say the Indian Scriptures. Christians who cannot imagine a higher destiny than eternal confinement in a little body would do well to meditate on the parable of the mustard seed, which Jesus likened to the kingdom of heaven. The mustard seed, Jesus said, though tiny, grows eventually to become a tree, "so that the birds of the air come and lodge in its branches." (Matthew 13:32.) Even so, the soul in communion with the Lord expands to embrace the infinity of consciousness that is God.

And Christians who imagine themselves *inherently* sinful, rather than sinning due to delusion, would do well to meditate on the parable of the prodigal son, whose *true* home was in God; and (if they aspire to heaven) on these words of Jesus, "No man hath ascended up to heaven, but he that came down from heaven." (John 3:13.)

34

Kriya Yoga

"BLESSED ARE THE PURE in heart, for they shall see God." The truth in these simple words has been acclaimed equally by great saints of East and West. It is a truth which every devotee would do well to ponder, for in all religions it is a common delusion to believe that mere affiliation with a body of worshippers will be one's passport to salvation. Yet Jesus didn't say, "Blessed are my followers, for they shall see God." His message was universal: By the yardstick of inner purity alone is a person's closeness to God determined.

How, then, can one achieve such purity? Is self-effort the answer? Is grace? St. Paul said, "By grace are ye saved through faith; and that not of yourselves; it is the gift of God: not of works, lest any man should boast."* Fundamentalist Christians often quote this passage as an argument against self-effort of any kind, and particularly against the practices of yoga. But the Book of Revelation states, "And, behold, I come quickly, and my reward is with me, *to give every man according as his work shall be.*"† Do these Scriptures contradict one another? Not at all.

St. Paul didn't mean that self-effort is futile, but only that God is above bargaining. But as for those inner efforts which lift the soul Godward, these are essential, else the Scriptures were written in vain.

To develop love for God, the first prerequisite is that no other desire hinder its free flow. This, then, is our first spiritual "work": to give up every desire that conflicts with our devotion. We need not *destroy* our desires so much as rechannel their energies Godward.

And it is in this true labor of love that the techniques of yoga serve most effectively. Wrong desires, it need hardly be added, could never be transmuted by technique alone. But just as the techniques of running are useful to those with a desire to be good runners, so the techniques of yoga can help devotees to control their physical energies, and to redirect them toward God. Yoga practice by itself won't give us God, but it *can* help us very much in our efforts to *give ourselves* to Him. The yoga science, in other words, helps us to *cooperate* with divine grace.

Take a simple example. Devotees naturally want to love God. Many, however, have no clear notion of how to go about loving Him. Too often their efforts are merely cerebral, and end in frustration. Yet Jesus hinted at a *technique* when he said, "Blessed are the pure in heart." For, as everyone who has loved deeply knows, it is in the *heart* that love is felt—not in the physical heart, literally, but in the *heart center*, or spinal nerve plexus just behind the heart. Christian saints have stressed again and again "the love of the *heart*." And yogis claim that love is developed more easily if, instead of merely *thinking* love, one will direct the thought of love upwards from the heart center, through the spine to the brain.

Thus, by its application of laws governing man's physical body and nervous system, the science of yoga helps one to become more

*Ephesians 2:8, 9.

†Revelation 22:12; italics mine.

receptive to the flow of divine grace, much as technical proficiency at the piano makes possible the uninterrupted flow of musical inspiration.

Likes and dislikes, and their resultant desires and aversions, are the root cause of mortal bondage.

Spiritual awakening takes place when *all* one's energy is directed upward to the spiritual eye. Hence the saying of Jesus, "Thou shalt love the Lord thy God with all thy *strength*": that is, "with all thy *energy*." This upward flow is obstructed by likes and dislikes.

Of all yoga techniques, the most effective, according to Paramhansa Yogananda, because the most central in its application, is Kriya Yoga. Kriya Yoga directs energy lengthwise around the spine, gradually neutralizing the eddies of likes and dislikes, and thereby freeing the soul. Of all the techniques of yoga, Kriya is quite probably the most ancient.

Yogananda often said that Kriya Yoga strengthens one in whatever path—whether devotion, discrimination, or service; Hindu, Christian, Moslem, or Judaic—one is inclined by temperament, or by upbringing, to follow.

"I wasn't sent to the West," Yogananda often told his audiences, "by Christ and the great masters of India to dogmatize you with a new theology. Jesus himself asked Babaji to send someone here to teach you the science of Kriya Yoga, that people might learn how to commune with God directly. I want to help you to attain actual experience of Him, through your daily practice of Kriya Yoga."

He added, "The time for knowing God has come!"

35

The Monks

IT OFTEN HAPPENS on the path that selfish desires spring up with surprising vigor out of the subconsciousness, to attack one's devotion. I've never seen such desires, when followed *as an alternative* to serving God selflessly, lead to anything but disappointment in the end.

Fortunate are those who, having realized their mistake, abandon it and return resolutely to the divine search. I have often admired one such devotee who, when others asked her how she dared to show herself at Mt. Washington again having once left it, replied joyously, "Do you expect me to worship my mistakes?"

Devotion is the greatest protection against delusion. But that devotee can hardly be found whose devotion *never* wanes, who never experiences times of spiritual emptiness or dryness, or never feels the tug of worldly desire. What is one to do when what Master called the "karmic bombs" of restlessness and desire strike, particularly in the midst of a dry period? In preparation against such a time, it is important to fortify oneself with regular habits of meditation, and with loyalty to one's chosen path. Once the habit of daily meditation becomes firmly established, one will cruise steadily through many a storm, succumbing neither to despondency when the way seems hard, nor to over-elation when it seems easy.

"Loyalty is the first law of God," Yogananda said. His reference was to that calm acceptance of one's own path which admits of no change of heart, which cannot be swayed by any obstacles on the way.

Loyalty, devotion, regular meditation, attunement with the guru—armed with these, every devotee can win the battle—not easily, perhaps, but in the end gloriously. The difference between those who stayed in the ashram and those who left it seemed to boil down to two alternatives: the desire to live only for God, and the desire to cling still to the little, human self. Jesus said, "Whosoever will save his life shall lose it." Leaving the ashram did not, of course, in itself constitute a fall, spiritually. Nor was such a fall, when it occurred, necessarily permanent for this lifetime. It all depended on whether one still put God first in one's life, and on whether one refused to accept even the severest setback as a final defeat. Whatever the circumstances, however, it was an unwise disciple who thought he could leave the ashram with impunity, certain that he would never forget God. "Delusion has its own power," Master warned us.

During the last two years of his life he spent many hours with the monks, teaching and inspiring them.

"Each of you must individually make love to God," he told us one evening. "Keep your mind at the Christ center when you work. Many come here, then talk and joke all the time—and play the organ." Master glanced meaningly at one of the monks. "They won't get God that way! There are mice living in the canyon on this property, but they are not developing spiritually! They haven't God. Don't think you can make spiritual progress merely by living here. You yourself must make the effort. Each of you stands alone before God."

Often he urged us to be steadfast in our practice of Kriya Yoga. "Practice Kriya night and day. It is the greatest key to salvation. Other people go by books and outer disciplines, but it will take them incarnations to reach God that way. Kriya is the geatest way of destroying temptation. Once you can feel the inner joy it gives you, no evil will be able to touch you. It will seem like stale cheese, then, compared with nectar. When others are idly talking or passing time, *you* go out into the garden and do a few Kriyas. What more do you need? Kriya will give you everything you are looking for. Practice it faithfully night and day."

"Sir," one of the disciples addressed him one afternoon, "How can one become more humble?"

"Humility," Master replied, "comes from seeing God as the Doer, not yourself. Seeing that, how can you feel proud for anything you have accomplished? Humility lies in the heart. It is not a show put on to impress others. Whatever you may be doing, tell yourself constantly, 'God is doing all this through me.' "

One of the disciples was being tormented by self-doubt. "As long as you are making the effort," Master consoled him, "God will *never* let you down!"

I asked Master one day, "Sir, in what way ought one to love people?"

"You should love God first," he replied, "then with His love, love others. In loving people for themselves, rather than as manifestations of God, you might get attached."

Speaking of love another time, he told us, "Human love is possessive and personal. Divine love is always impersonal. To develop devotion in the right way, and to protect it from the taint of possessive, personal love, it is better not to seek God above all for His love until one is highly developed. Seek Him first of all for His bliss."

"Never count your faults," he once told us. "Be concerned only that you love God enough. And," he added, "don't tell your faults to others, lest someday in a fit of anger they hold them against you. But tell your faults to God. From Him you should try to conceal nothing."

The American "go-getter" spirit drew praise from him. " 'Eventually? Eventually? Why not now!' *That* is the American way that I like. Seek God with that kind of determination and you will surely find Him!"

Many hours he spent talking with us, giving us help and encouragement. Above all he urged us to seek our inspiration inwardly, in meditation.

Hearing one of the monks chanting in the main chapel one

evening, to the accompaniment of an Indian harmonium, he paused during the course of a conversation downstairs. Blissfully, then, he remarked, "That is what I like to hear in this hermitage of God!"

36

The Wave
And The Ocean

"DIVINE MOTHER ONCE SAID to me, 'Those to whom I give too much, I do not give Myself.'" Master was explaining to us the difference between joyous acceptance of divine favors, vouchsafed by God as a sign of His love, and a desire for the favors themselves.

"Seek God for Himself," he told us, "not for any gift that He might give you." Unlike many proponents of spiritual "new thought," he taught us that the true test of spirituality is indifference to everything but God's love. To make religion a matter of "manifesting" an endless succession of worldly goods would be, he implied, to make a religion of materialism. The sincere devotee prefers rather to "manifest" a simple life. All that he owns he considers God's property altogether, to be returned joyously to its Owner at a moment's notice.

Master used to say, "Whenever I see somebody who needs something of mine more than I do, I give it away."

"A few years ago," he told us, "I had a fine musical instrument, an esraj from India. I loved to play devotional music on it. But a visitor one day admired it. Unhesitatingly I gave it to him. Years later someone asked me, 'Weren't you just a *little* sorry?' 'Never for a moment!' I replied. Sharing one's happiness with others only expands one's own happiness."

Master kept only enough money personally to finance his trips to the different ashrams. Even this amount he often gave away.

He displayed the same indifference to all outward enjoyments. It wasn't apathy; enthusiasm for all aspects of life was a hallmark of his personality. But it was clear that he enjoyed things not for their own sake, but because they manifested in various ways his one, infinite Beloved.

Great masters have the power to assume others' karma, much as a strong man might take onto his own body blows intended for a weaker person. Occasionally—especially toward the end of their lives, to help their disciples through years without the guru's physical presence—they assume large amounts of karma. At such times their own bodies may suffer temporarily.

It was such a gift that Master now bestowed on us. The result was that, for a time, he couldn't walk.

But he remarked smiling, "This body is not everything. Some people have feet, but can't walk all over!"

One afternoon I was helping him into his car. "You are getting better, Sir," I exclaimed thankfully.

"Who is getting better?" Master's tone was impersonal.

"I meant your body, Sir."

"What's the difference? The wave protruding from the ocean bosom is still a part of the ocean. This is God's body. If He wants to make it well, all right. If He wants to keep it unwell, all right. It is best to remain impartial. If you have health and are attached to it, you will always be afraid of losing it. And if you are attached to good health and become ill, you will be always grieving for the good that you have lost.

"Man's greatest trouble is egoism, the consciousness of individuality. He takes everything that happens to him as affecting *him*, personally. Why be affected? You are not this body. You are *He!* Everything is Spirit."

One evening, speaking of his illness, he said, "It was nothing! When the wisdom dinner from the plate of life has been eaten, it no longer matters whether you keep the plate, or break it and throw it away.

"Man was put here on earth to seek God. That is the only reason for his existence. Friends, job, material interests: All these by themselves mean nothing."

"Sir," one of the monks inquired, "is it wrong to ask God for material things?"

"It is all right, if you need them," Master replied. "But you should always say, 'Give me this or that, *provided* it is all right with you.' Many of the things people want would prove harmful to them if they got them. Leave it to God to decide what you ought to have."

Whatever Master's topic of conversation—whether some aspect of the spiritual path, or some perfectly ordinary task that he wanted done—if one "listened" sensitively enough one always felt a subtle power emanating from him. If one took this awareness within, one felt blessed with a heightened sense of joy and freedom.

"Is this work a new religion?" I asked him one day.

"It is a new *expression*," he corrected me.

Truth is one: *Sanatan Dharma* as it is known in India—"the Eternal Religion." The great world religions are all branches on that single tree.

Sectarianism is divisive. "The one Ocean has become all its waves," Master told me once, when I questioned him about his own role in the religious evolution of this planet. "You should look to the Ocean, not to the little waves protruding on its bosom."

37

Reminiscences

"I N THE EARLY DAYS of Mt. Washington, a visitor once inquired superciliously, 'What are the assets of this organization?'

" 'None!' I replied. 'Only God.' "

Master was reminiscing about his early years in America. Toward the end of his life, in addition to counseling us, he spent many hours trying to make us feel a part of that long period of his life before most of us had come to him.

"My reply on that occasion was literally true, too," Master chuckled. "We hadn't *any* money! But it would be just as true today, when our work is financially strong. For our strength has always been God alone. We might lose everything materially speaking, and in His love we would still possess all that really mattered.

"Years ago a rich man came here who thought to buy me with his wealth. Knowing we badly needed money just then, he tried in certain ways to get me to compromise my ideals. I refused. Finally he said, 'You'll starve because you didn't listen.' Leaving here, he talked against me to a rich acquaintance of his, a student of this work. And *that* was the man God chose to give us the help we needed!

"He is happiest who gives everything to God." Master told an amusing story to illustrate his own preference for simple living, free of all ostentation.

"A wealthy student of mine wanted to buy me a new overcoat. Taking me into a well-known clothing store, he invited me to select any coat that I wanted. Seeing one that looked nice, I reached out for it. But then, seeing the price tag, I quickly withdrew my hand. It was a very expensive coat.

" 'But I'd be *happy* to buy it for you,' my friend insisted. He added an expensive hat to match. I appreciated his kindness in giving me these gifts. But whenever I wore them, I felt uncomfortable. Expensive possessions are a responsibility.

" 'Divine Mother,' I finally prayed, 'this coat is too good for me. Please take it away.'

"Soon afterwards I was scheduled to lecture in Trinity Auditorium. I sensed that the coat would be taken away from me that evening, so I emptied the pockets. After the lecture the coat was gone. What a relief!

"But then I spotted an omission. 'Divine Mother,' I prayed, 'You forgot to take the hat!'

"You don't have to *own* a thing to enjoy it," Master told us. "To possess things is all right, provided your possessions don't possess you, but ownership often means only added worries. It is much better to own everything in God, and not to cling to anything with the ego."

Master told us of a time when his nonattachment had been tested. "I was standing alone one evening on a dark street corner in New York, when three hold-up men came up from behind me, one of them pointing a gun.

" 'Give us your money,' they demanded.

" 'Here it is,' I said, not at all disturbed. 'But I want you to know that I am not giving it to you out of fear. I have such wealth in my heart that, by comparison, money means nothing to me.' They were so astonished! I then gazed at them with God's power. They burst into tears. Returning my money, they cried, 'We can't live this way any more!' Then, overwhelmed by the experience, they ran away."

Master usually accepted evil as a regrettable, but necessary, part of the cosmic drama. He fought it only in those who sought his spiritual aid. "The villain's role on the stage," he used to say, "is to get people to love the hero. Evil's role, similarly, in the drama of life is to spur people on to seek goodness." There were times, however, when he became an avenging angel, particularly when the lives of devotees were affected.

The mother of one close disciple was afflicted with cancer. Finding a sanatorium that advertised a supposedly miraculous cure, she entered it hopefully.

"All they gave their patients," Master told us, "was water! They took their money, fed them nothing, and simply waited for them to die. When I found out their scheme, I cried, 'Divine Mother, destroy that place!' Within a month the police came in and closed it. The leaders all went to prison."

No environment was without God to him. "Do you know where I wrote my poem, *'Samadhi'?*" he asked us one day. "It was on the New York subway! As I was writing, I rode back and forth from one end of the line to the other. No one asked for my ticket. In fact," he added with a twinkle, "no one saw me!"

Master often regaled us with amusing anecdotes. "Because of my robe and long hair, people sometimes thought I was a woman. Once, at a Boston flower exhibition, I wanted to find the men's room. A guard directed me to a certain door. Trustingly I went in. My goodness! Ladies to the left of me, ladies to the right of me, ladies everywhere! I rushed out, and once more approached the guard.

" 'I want the *men's* room,' I insisted. Eyeing me suspiciously, he pointed to another door. This time as I entered a man cried out, 'Not in here, lady! Not in here!'

"In a basso profundo voice I answered, 'I know what I am doing!'

"When I first came to America," he continued, "my father used to send me money. But I wanted to rely wholly on God, so I returned it. In the beginning God let me taste a little hardship, to test my faith in Him, but my faith was firm, and He never failed me."

To Master, human experience was, in a sense, part of a process of divine healing. Man's supreme disease, he said, is spiritual ignorance. Though the supreme "cure" he offered was divine bliss, he healed many physical ailments.

One such healing occurred years before I entered the work. Master told us the story:

"It was during the Chicago World's Fair, in 1933. Dr. Lewis telephoned me in Los Angeles to report that a friend of his had a blood clot on the heart, and was dying. Could I help him? I sat in meditation and prayed. Suddenly a great power went out from me, like an explosion. In that same instant the man, who had been in a coma, was healed. A nurse was in the room with him—not a spiritual woman at all. She testified later that she'd heard an explosion in the room, and seen a brilliant flash of light. The man at once sat up, completely recovered."

Master then spoke of the most important kind of healing: the dispelling of soul ignorance. "That is why we have these ashrams," he said, "for those who want to give their lives to God, to be healed of *all* suffering forevermore." He talked on about those earlier years. Looking at us sweetly, he concluded, "How I wish you all had been with me then! So many years had to pass before you came."

38

His Last Days

DURING THE LAST year and a half of Master's life, long-time disciples gathered around him, as though somehow aware that his end was approaching. Some who, for a variety of reasons, had not seen him for years, visited him now. Others who hadn't met him yet, but whose destiny it was to meet him in this life, came, as if hurrying to get in before it was too late.

We all felt that the time was fast approaching when Master would leave this world. Master himself hinted as much. To Dr. Lewis he remarked one day, "We have lived a good life together. It seems only yesterday that we met. In a little while we shall be separated, but soon we'll be together again."

During his last months, especially, he found his greatest earthly joy in those disciples who had lived up to his divine expectations of them. Often he praised Saint Lynn, Sister Gyanamata, Daya Mata, and others.

"Sir," I said to Master one day, "after you are gone, will you be as near to us as you are now?"

"To those who *think* me near," he replied, "I will be near."

Several days before the end, a disciple asked, "Have all your disciples of this life come yet, Sir?"

"I am waiting for two or three more," Master replied.

He had been staying at his Twenty-Nine Palms retreat. He returned to Mt. Washington on March 2nd to meet His Excellency, Binay R. Sen, India's recently appointed Ambassador to the United States. On the evening of his return, he embraced each of us lovingly, and blessed us. To some he gave words of personal help, to others, encouragement to be stable in their efforts, to still others the advice to meditate more. Afterwards I got to see him briefly upstairs, alone.

Many times over the past three and a half years Master had scolded me, mostly for my slowness in understanding him perfectly, sometimes for not weighing in advance the possible consequences of my words. I knew that he often said, "I scold only those who listen, not those who don't," but in my heart there lingered a certain hurt. Try as I would, I couldn't rationalize it away. For months I had been hungering for a few words of approval from him.

Now, alone with me, he gazed into my eyes with deep love and understanding, and said, "You have pleased me very much. I want you to know that." What a burden lifted from my heart at these few, simple words!

On Tuesday, March 4th, the Ambassador and his party visited Mt. Washington. I served Master and his guests upstairs. During their visit Mr. Ahuja, India's Consul-General in San Francisco, remarked to Master, "Ambassadors may come, and ambassadors may go. You, Paramhansaji, are India's real Ambassador to America."

Thursday evening, March 6th, Master returned from a ride in the car. The monks had just finished their group practice of the energization exercises. As we gathered around him, he touched each of us in blessing. He then spoke at length about some of the delusions devotees encounter on the path.

"Don't waste your time," he said. "No one can give you the desire for God. That is something you must cultivate yourself.

"Why waste your spiritual perceptions? When you have filled the bucket of your consciousness with the milk of peace, keep it that way; don't drive holes in it with joking and idle speech.

"Don't waste time on distractions—reading all the time and so on. If reading is instructive, of course it is good. But I tell people, 'If you read one hour, then write two hours, think three hours, and meditate all the time.' No matter how much this organization keeps me busy, I never forego my daily tryst with God."

The following day, March 7th, he was scheduled to attend a banquet at the Biltmore Hotel in honor of the Indian Ambassador. "Imagine!" he said, "I've taken a room at the Biltmore. That's where I first started in this city!"

Master had asked me to attend the banquet with Dick Haymes, the popular singer and movie actor. Dick had recently become a disciple, and had taken Kriya initiation from me.

Years ago Master had said, "When I leave this earth, I want to go speaking of my America and my India." And in a song about India that he had written, to the tune of the popular song, "My California," he paraphrased the ending of that popular version with the words, "I know when I die, in joy I will sigh for my sunny, grand old India!" Once, too, in a lecture he had stated, "A heart attack is the easiest way to die. That is how *I* choose to die." This evening, all these predictions were to prove true.

Master was scheduled to speak after the banquet. His brief talk was so sweet, so almost tender, that I think everyone present felt embraced in the gossamer net of his love. Warmly he spoke of India and America, and of their respective contributions to world peace and true human progress. He talked of their future cooperation. Finally he read his beautiful poem, "My India."

Throughout his speech I was busy recording his words, keeping my eyes on my notebook. He came to the last lines of the poem:

Where Ganges, woods, Himalayan caves and men dream God.

I am hallowed; my body touched that sod!

"Sod" became a long-drawn sigh. Suddenly from all sides of the room there was a shriek. I looked up.

"What is it?" I demanded of Dick Haymes, seated beside me. "What happened?"

"Master fainted," he replied.

Oh, no, Master! You wouldn't faint. You've left us. You've left us!

They brought Master's body to Mt. Washington and placed it lovingly on his bed. One by one we went in and knelt by his bedside.

"How many thousands of years it took," marveled an older

disciple, gazing upon him in quiet awe, "to produce such a perfect face!"

Later on, after we'd left the room, Daya Mata remained alone with Master's body. As she gazed at him, a tear formed on his left eyelid, and slowly trickled down his cheek.Lovingly she caught it with her handkerchief.

In death, as in life, he was telling his beloved disciple, and through her the rest of us, "I love you always, through endless cycles of time, unconditionally, without any desire except fot *your* happiness, forever, in God!"

Part III

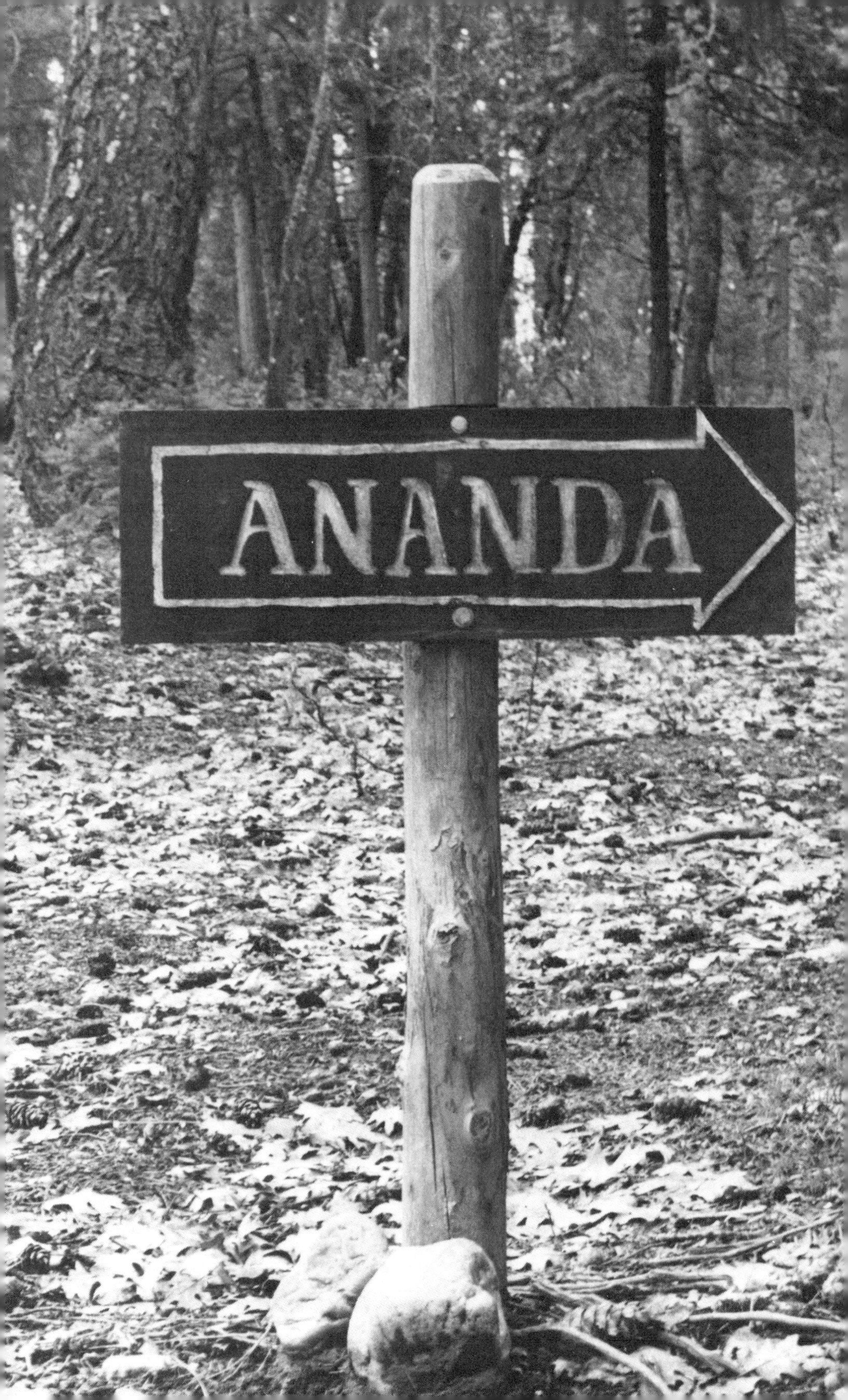
ANANDA

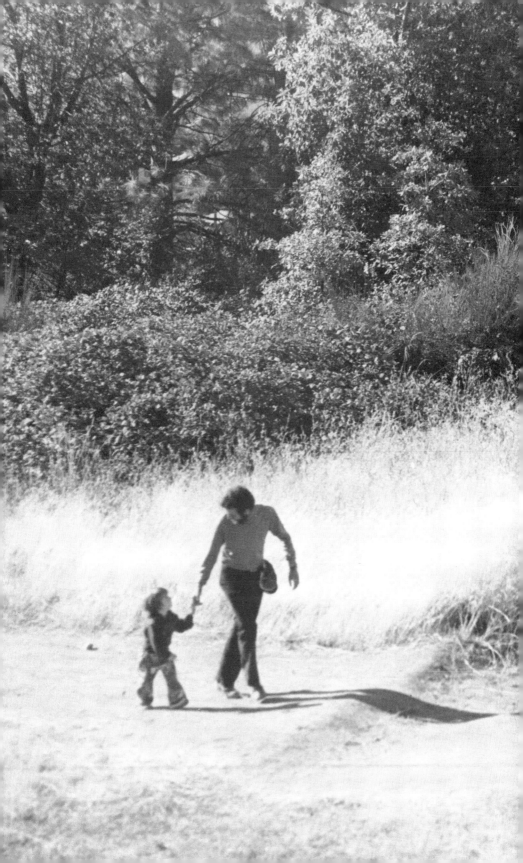

Ananda means joy . . .

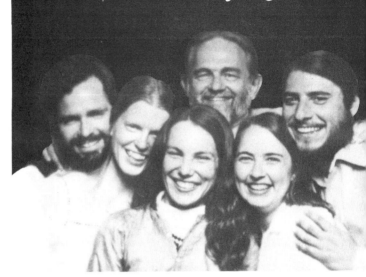

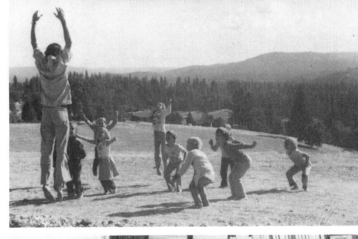

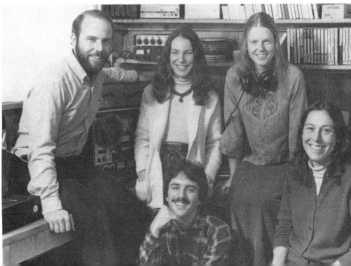

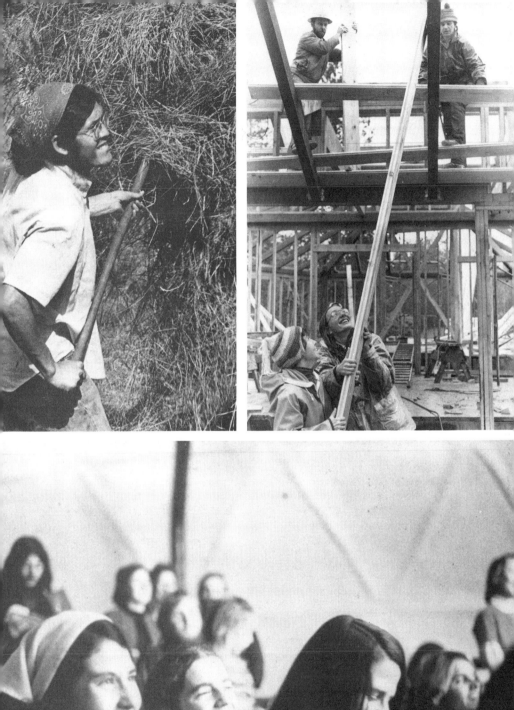
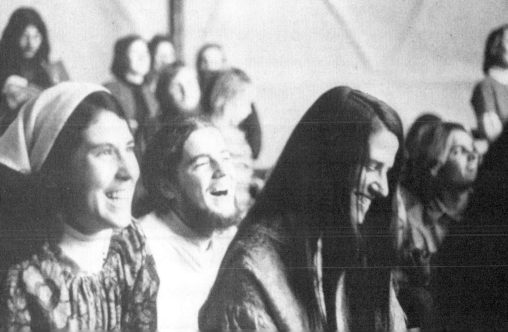

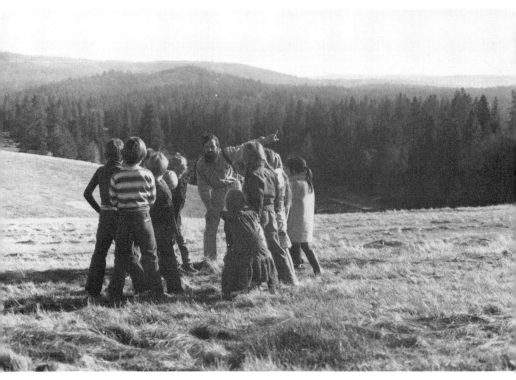

33

Ananda member Joseph Bharat Cornell, author of *Sharing Nature With Children*, leads some of our children in one of the games from his popular book.

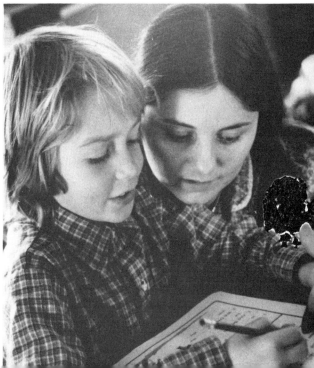

34

Sasha, one of Ananda's 70 students, receives from teacher Mary Kieran the personalized attention that is essential to Ananda's How-to-Live system of instruction. Ananda's schools are based on the educational methods of Paramhansa Yogananda.

How-to-Live Schools

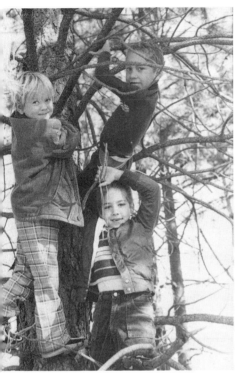

35

Who needs a Jungle gym when he can climb a tree?

36

How-to-Live education, in addition to academics, includes training in moral and spiritual values: cooperation with others, and careful cultivation of the life in oneself, and in the world around one.

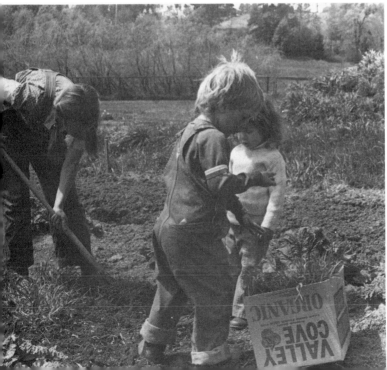

Ananda Guest Programs

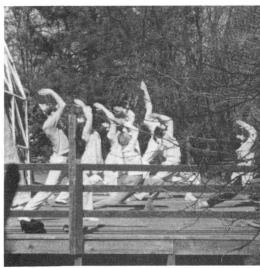

37

Ananda Meditation Retreat offers hundreds of visitors a year a chance to receive meditative, spiritual, and "how-to-live" teachings.

38

"I am joyful, I am free!" Retreatants greet the day with yoga postures on the temple deck.

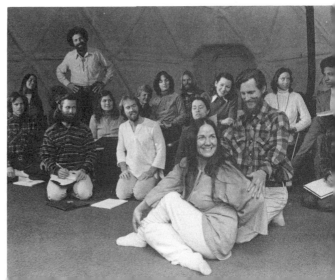

39

Students attend Ananda's Yoga Teachers Training Course from around the world.

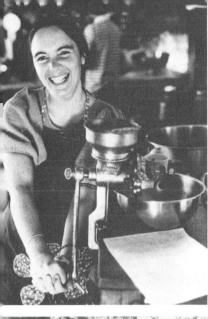

40

Gourmet vegetarian meals are prepared at the Retreat. Much of the food is grown in our own garden.

41

In summer classes and services are often held out-of-doors in the Temple of Leaves.

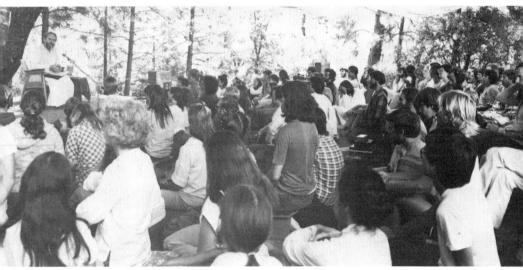

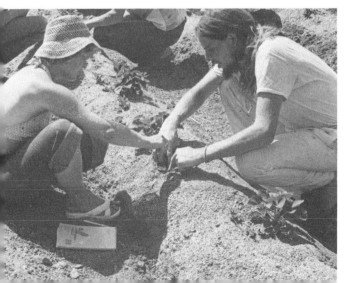

42

Ananda's apprenticeship program is designed to give guests a chance to learn important skills while living and working in the community.

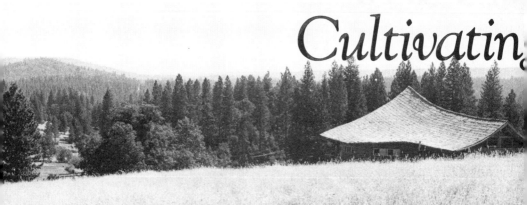

Cultivating

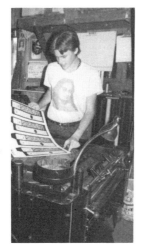

43

I designed our Ananda
Publications building to
express in architecture
Ananda's aspiration to soar
outward over the hearts of
men and upward toward
God.

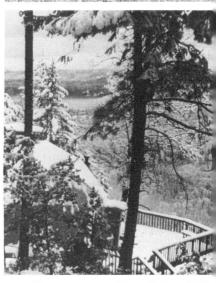

44

My home at Ayodhya, our monastery, is
alternately where I spend time in seclusion
and where I render grateful service through
writing, recording, and teaching.

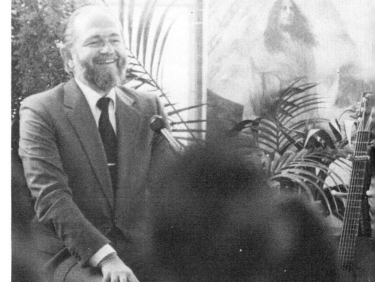

45

A busy schedule has
taken me to many parts
of the world.

Master's Garden of Souls

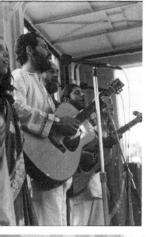

46

People across the country have heard the Ananda Singers render my Songs of Divine Joy.

What is love?
Is it only ours?
Or does love whisper in the flowers?
Surely we, children of this world,
Could not love by our own powers.

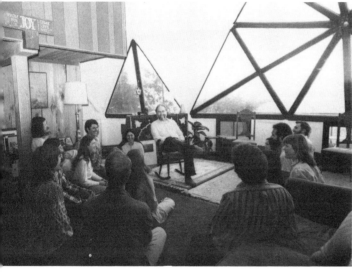

47

An informal spiritual gathering in my home.

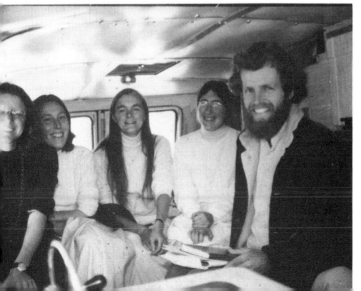

48

The people at Ananda seem to me embodiments, truly, of Babaji's words to Sri Yukteswar in *Autobiography of a Yogi:* "I perceive potential saints in America and Europe, waiting to be awakened."

Ever-Widening Circle

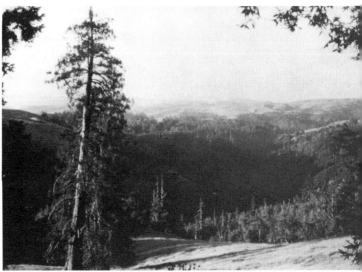

49

Ananda comprises also
six subsidiary communi-
ties in San Francisco,
Atherton, Stockton,
Sacramento, Nevada
City and this one:
Ocean Song, a 900-acre
farm, school and
projected healing center
near Bodega Bay, north
of San Francisco.

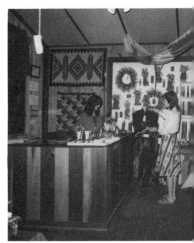

50

Mountain Song in Nevada City, one
of Ananda's over 30 supportive
businesses, carries hand-crafted
items, many of them by craftspeople
of the area.

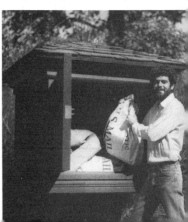

51

People write to Ananda from all
over the world. First stop for their
letters: our "dog house" mailbox at
the entrance way to the farm.

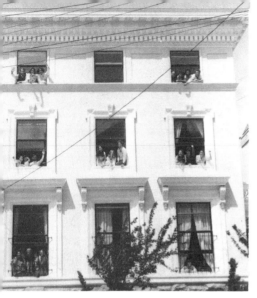

52

Ananda House in San Francisco is a forty-five-room mansion at 2320 Broadway overlooking the bay. Members live here, conduct services and classes in and around San Francisco, and operate Earthsong, a beautiful cafe and book store in the city's Sunset district.

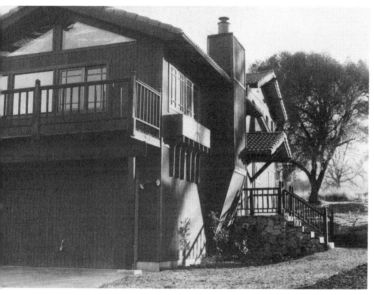

53

Ananda Construction Company builds quality homes throughout northern California.

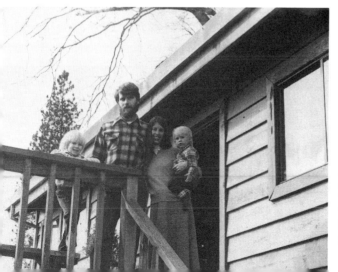

54

One of the fundamental needs of our age is for putting down roots again. We have extended ourselves too far outward, away from the Self within, and away from the natural rhythms of the planet on which we live. Ananda strives to demonstrate the truth of Yogananda's words, "Simplicity of living plus high thinking lead to the greatest happiness."

39

My Words Are
in the Ether!

I SPENT A TOTAL of fourteen years in Self-Realization Fellowship, ten of them at Mt. Washington, and four more with Yogoda Satsanga Society, SRF's Indian affiliate. In 1962 Master took me out of his organization, though not out of his work, to devote myself to the service for which he had trained me. Since then I have written books, lectured widely, and founded Ananda Village, a flourishing community near Nevada City, California. For all of these activities, the relative freedom of private, rather than institutional, life proved, in the beginning at least, a necessity. Thousands have been brought to Master's teachings who might, otherwise, never have realized that in the techniques he taught, and in the answers he gave to life's problems, lay the path they themselves were seeking.

Perhaps in all of these activities, but certainly in the founding of
Ananda, Master's charge to me of a "great work" has been fulfilled.
Ananda Village, with its hundreds of members, is one of the most
successful "new-age" communities in the world. Visitors come from
many countries, both for spiritual inspiration and to study how to
found successful communities themselves.

Frequently, now, when people seek my advice on founding
communities, I urge them to seek Paramhansa Yogananda's
blessings. I hope I am not guilty of sectarianism in so doing, for one
of the most refreshing aspects of his teachings is their resolute non-
sectarianism. Yet it was Yogananda who brought this communitarian
way of life to the world in this age—who in a very real sense set the
stamp of his spiritual power on the success of this ideal. As he put it:
"My spoken words are registered in the ether, in the spirit of God,
and they shall move the West!" For the blessings he gave to this new
movement he may truly be called the "patron saint" of "world-
brotherhood colonies"—whether or not particular "colonies"
contain disciples of his path. Certainly, those communities which
have sought his blessings seem to have received a very special kind of
help.

My years with Master may be seen, in retrospect, as a training for
these subsequent years of service to him.

The position he put me in as head of the monks gave me invaluable
experience in organizing, leading, and counseling others. So also did
my years in the ministry, and working in the main office of SRF.

In 1952 I was given the job of reorganizing that main office, at Mt.
Washington. A year later I became the director of SRF Center
activities around the world, and, in 1955, the main minister of our
church in Hollywood. In 1960 I was appointed the first vice-
president of SRF and of YSS, and a member of both Boards of
Directors.

All of these activities helped prepare me for the work of founding
Ananda.

In addition, my years in India from 1958 to 1962, teaching and
lecturing to thousands around the country, prepared me in another
way: They enabled me to understand Master's teachings in an
Eastern, as well as in a Western, context. The insights gained thereby
enabled me to bridge the gap between these dissimilar cultures, and
to demonstrate how each—especially the Indian and the American—
was uniquely in a position to help the other.

In August, 1955, I took final vows of renunciation in solemn ceremony, receiving *sannyas* (ordination into full monkhood) from Sri Daya Mata, the third President of Self-Realization Fellowship. On this occasion I was formally given the name Kriyananda (meaning "divine bliss through Kriya Yoga," and, alternatively, "divine bliss in action"). As a *sannyasi*, now, my official title became, in the ancient Indian tradition (with which SRF is officially aligned), *Swami.*

My separation from SRF in 1962 was far from easy, both for me and for SRF. But it was necessary as a means of freeing me, at least for a time, to concentrate on the work that I had to do. The mechanics of that separation no longer matter now. Indeed, my hope is that Ananda and SRF will someday unite. For the two are devoted to the same path, and to the same basic ideals. Meanwhile, I am happy to say, unity of spirit has always existed. The members of Ananda Village are required to be SRF members also. They accept Paramhansa Yogananda as their guru, and the SRF President as his highest representative in his work.

40

I Do Battle
with Meaninglessness

N JUNE, 1962, I read an article in SPAN, the American Government magazine in India. Its author, the head of the philosophy department at M.I.T., discussed the influence of science on modern philosophical thought. The leading thinkers of our times, according to him, are basically nihilistic; they consider the universe completely meaningless. Evolution, to them, is accidental; it has no conscious direction. Human values are irrelevant, except as a purely social convenience; they have no foundation in objective reality. The general scheme of things is irrational; reason itself is but a subjective, human effort to impose meaning on universal Chaos.

How, I asked myself, had intelligent, presumably thoughtful human beings brought themselves to such a moral impasse? Trained as I was in the subtleties of Vedanta philosophy, I could see clearly that the problem was not actually born of scientific revelation. Old values had not been destroyed by science. All that had been lost was old *definitions* of those values.

I longed for the opportunity to study these problems, and to do battle with obvious misconceptions which were, it was clear to me, the greatest single threat to mankind in this century. For what molds man, and determines his destiny, is not his objective realities, but his inner *response* to them, his subjective world of ideas.

I longed, as I say, for the opportunity to study these problems, and to write about them. But how could I ever do so, engaged as I was with the more immediate problems of the SRF organization? On a subtle level of awareness it seemed to me (though I rejected the thought consciously) that the time had come for a change in my work, that Master now wanted me to do the task for which he had prepared me. The reason I rejected this thought was that years of serving my guru within the framework of his organization had conditioned me to *equate* him with his organization. But in time I faced the question: What was he himself trying to do? Then I understood that what service to him really meant to me was making his teachings better known.

It was he who solved this dilemma for me, long before I myself understood the solution, by taking me out of SRF.

In September, 1962, I settled in northern California. There I devoted myself to years of research in a variety of fields. I lived for six months in a Roman Catholic hermitage, studying the writings and sayings of great Christian saints, and pondering the numerous links which this study enabled me to discover between their insights and those of India's great yogis. I studied the findings of modern science, and pondered how to bridge the gap between Twentieth Century materialism and the subtle, spiritual realities of which I found more than a hint in the annals of physics, chemistry, and biology.

"People are so skillful in their ignorance!" Master had exclaimed. I set myself the task now of sparring with that ignorance, and of turning it, wherever possible, to spiritual advantage.

The fruits of this study found their way eventually into a book that I titled *Crises in Modern Thought*. They also found their way into my lectures and classes, which were increasingly in demand over a considerable area.

I wrote songs, too, hoping through music to touch people's hearts in a way that mere words might never do. Most of these songs expressed a philosophy of joy. After the first album of them came out in 1965, people who had ordered it from across the country wrote to say that the songs gave them renewed hope in life.

In addition I authored other books. I saw all these works as comprising the spokes of a wheel, each of them radiating outward from a hub of divine truth into different, and in some cases quite varied, fields of human interest.

For five years I prepared myself philosophically, as earlier I had done organizationally, for the even more demanding task that still lay ahead of me: that of founding the first of Master's "world-brotherhood colonies." For years I had studied the problem of how to found a successful community. I had read histories of past communities; visited currently functioning communities in various parts of the world; talked to economists, sociologists, and others who might shed light on this matter; and sought inner guidance in meditation. Always I was mindful of my silent vow to do everything in my power to fulfill Master's "world-brotherhood colony" dream.

From 1965 onwards, also, though aware that the time was not yet ripe, I followed every clue that might lead to the eventual purchase of land for such a community.

In 1967, finally, I found the land that was to be the starting point for Ananda.

41

Land Ho!

I KNEW WITHIN MINUTES that it was the land I had been seeking. Lovely, wooded terrain, 3,000 feet high in the foothills of the Sierra Nevada of northern California, it was situated about twenty miles north of the little former mining town of Nevada City. The property was remote, the approach road deeply rutted by rain, and passable only on foot. There wasn't a house within miles. The property hadn't even a spring. But I felt Master's blessings there, and his inner guidance to begin Ananda.

For some months, as if in anticipation of this next step, my income had been increasing. More students were attending my classes. The Peace Corps had invited me to head their cultural indoctrination program for a group of students being sent to India. I had no wealthy sponsors, but God made it possible for me to earn all the money I needed.

To tell the truth, my first dream was of a place of seclusion for myself. On a deeper level of awareness I knew this was little more than a dream, that what I was being called to found was a community. But, both because my personal desire was for a hermitage for myself, and because I wanted to be sure of being truly guided in any effort to build an outward work, I deliberately resisted at first the communitarian aspect of this project. If, I reasoned, Master did indeed want me to found a community, he would find ways of forcing events so that one happened.

He found ways all right. Until I resigned myself to building Ananda, all my efforts to build a private hermitage for myself were resolutely thwarted.

I find that, somehow, I have always lived my life on two levels: a conscious level, on which I approach things according to my own personal inclinations; and another one, more dimly perceived, on which I seem to know how things are going to have to be whether I want them that way or not. I had this inner knowledge where the present project was concerned. Nevertheless, as I set myself to building my own hermitage, I should have listened to that soft inner whisper. It told me from the start that I had made the wrong choice, and that if the rest of the project was to develop in the right way I would have to think of myself last, not first.

"But all I want," I told myself, "is a place to seek God. What's so selfish about that?" If I'd waited for an answer, the rest of the year might have gone more smoothly for me.

As a structure for my home, I had decided on a dome. The idea had first come to me in India, in 1961. There my plan had been to build a temple; my meditations had suggested this type of structure to my mind as the most conducive to inner calmness and expansion. What I envisioned at that time was a hemisphere coming down on all sides to about eye level—more or less like the inside of a planetarium. A flat ceiling seemed to me to have the psychological, even psychic, effect of pressing down on the head. The high domes, on the other hand, that one finds in temples around the world suggest a heavenly state far removed from present human realities. For meditation, with the present inner peace that it induces, a dome that descended to eye level seemed ideal, as though harmonizing with nature and its round "inverted bowl" of the sky. The human head, too, is a kind of dome. Perhaps one reason it soothes one to be inside a dome is that the rays of energy going outward from the brain are echoed back most harmoniously from the inner surface of a similar structure. After returning from India I visited a planetarium, and was interested to discover that even with children squirming and giggling all around me, and while people were still entering and the lights still on, a distinct impression of peace emanated from that interior.

I wanted, as I say, to construct a perfect dome. But inquiries convinced me that the cost would be prohibitive. Then one day a student in one of my classes introduced me to a concept that was new to me: the geodesic dome, an invention of Buckminster Fuller. For me, this was a compromise. "Bucky's" straight lines and flat planes produce a marvel of engineering, but esthetically they conflict with the roundness of a true hemisphere. Still, it was the closest thing to a possibility that I had come upon so far. I resolved to follow in the footsteps of Buckminster Fuller.

It was easier resolved than done. No one seemed to know the mathematical formulae. One company that I found made domes, but were tool designers, not architects; their squat structures reminded me of toadstools out of a book of nursery rhymes. This, I decided, was just too much of a compromise.

At last Charles Tart, a professor at the University of California at Davis, showed me a geodesic dome that he was constructing in his back yard. It was called a "sun dome." Inexpensive, beautiful in its simplicity, and easy for any amateur like me to construct, it offered me my first ray of real hope. I clutched it as eagerly (and as foolishly) as a drowning man would a straw.

Easy it may have been to construct, but building the platform, cutting the struts exactly to the required angles, assembling them into triangles, then covering them with plastic, required months of unceasing labor. After all my years of waiting, I was determined to build my retreat if possible that year.

No, Kriyananda, it was not to be. I got the dome up all right. The last triangle was about to go in, after which, supposedly, the dome would stand firm. But until it had been fully assembled, its strength was precarious.

Suddenly a strong gust of wind rushed up from the valley; the entire structure fell to the ground, a jumble of matchsticks and plastic.

Refusing to give up, I set out immediately to replace the broken pieces, reassembling all the triangles, and stapling them together with greater care than the first time. Weeks later, the new structure was up. It was, in all fairness, more beautiful than anything we have built since. Its delicate struts were an esthetic delight. But Keats was wrong: Beauty is not necessarily truth. The "sun dome" proved a snare and a delusion.

I did not realize that the planners had designed it to sit cozily in a fenced-in back yard, as Charlie Tart's was, well protected from strong winds, and preferably even from the mildest zephyr. Up on the hilltop at Ananda the late autumn winds can get up to sixty or seventy miles an hour. In the first storm we had, my beautiful dome-house simply disintegrated. I walked away from it without even looking back.

But after a few days I summoned the courage to try once again. This time, after re-cutting many more pieces and reassembling them, I screwed them all firmly together with large metal plates. This time, I was sure, no wind could possibly rip them apart. The wind didn't have to. Alas, I knew nothing of its power to lift a hemisphere, similar to the lift it exerts on the upper portion of the wing of an airplane. I returned to Ananda soon after I had put up my dome for the third time. I was eager, before winter descended in earnest, to get at least a little of that solitary meditation I had been planning for so long.

I arrived to find pieces of the dome draped artistically over the surrounding bushes. Worst of all, because this time the pieces had been screwed so firmly together, virtually every one of them was broken. There was nothing to do but recognize defeat, and accept it calmly. I sat down on the open platform, and, surprisingly perhaps, had a joyous meditation.

But to me it was a sign that I would not be able to have my own home until I had built a temple, and perhaps even a community, for the benefit of others.

42

Point Counterpoint

M Y HOME-TO-BE had blown down for the third time. I found myself almost without funds. There was no choice for me but to go back to teaching classes again. This I did intensively, traveling to a different city every evening, determined now to earn the money necessary to build a retreat for others as well as for myself. And as long as I was putting forth so much energy, I decided, if possible, also to take the first step toward building the cooperative community I had been contemplating.

To many people, my dream of starting a community was only that: a dream: impractical, visionary, an adolescent fancy doomed to ignoble failure. A professor at UC Davis did a study of communitarian ventures at about this time, and found that the average life expectancy of a new community was only thirty days! Clearly, the odds against our success were enormous.

The first, and forever greatest, obstacle proved to be that invariable stumbling block: human nature. In February, 1968, I invited people to a formal meeting to discuss plans for forming a cooperative community. I had planned to have only a few close friends and co-workers at this first meeting. Others, however, whom I hardly knew, but who claimed to be interested in the project, appeared also, uninvited. Their presence proved a mixed blessing.

"How do we know you're on the level?" one of them demanded.

"If you start something this big, you'll soon forget all about your ideal of serving people."

"I know a teacher who became involved in building a place similar to this. It took so much of his energy that he lost his inner peace, and today he's a MONSTER!"

"Think of it, everyone. If Kriyananda really wanted to draw us into this thing as partners, *why didn't he call this meeting sooner?*"

The only thing to do at this point was to serve tea and cookies.

But the meeting was not a total disaster. Realizing that by mere talk I would never be able to give people a clear picture of what I had in mind, I sat down at last with the gathered notes and reflections of many years, and wrote a book that, even today, stands alone in its field: *Cooperative Communities—How to Start Them, and Why.* After publishing it, first in looseleaf form, and distributing it to all who expressed an interest in the idea, I decided to give everyone time to reflect on it before broaching the subject again.

My own enthusiasm had led me to expect a quick, positive response from anyone to whom I described my ideas. I had overlooked the many years it had taken me to grow into them myself.

Many potentially interested persons, I now realized, needed not only enough time to reflect on these ideas, but also the reassurance of seeing something already solidly accomplished. It is one of the curious facts of human life that, for most ventures to be started, people are the prime necessity, but that, for most people to become involved at all, the venture itself must already be well under way.

No one, I decided, could accuse me of black motives if I built a meditation retreat. It was a project about which little theorizing was necessary, and it would attract active participation. Slowly, out of this group labor, the seeds might sprout that would grow in time to become the cooperative community.

I had reached the conclusion, by means which the tactful reader will doubtless fail to recognize, that I was not cut out to be a carpenter. The worst of it was that none of my friends were carpenters, either. But by this time I was earning a fair amount of money by teaching classes. Some money was coming in also from generous friends. This income, plus a few stocks that my father had given me over the years, totaled about sixteen thousand dollars— enough for me to consider hiring professional help.

I still wanted those geodesic domes. The only company that made them was still that one which manufactured pre-fabs vaguely reminiscent of toadstools. I bowed to the inevitable. At least these were something I could afford.

I found a carpenter who expressed confidence that he would be able to put up our buildings in two weeks. "Go ahead," I told him. Had I shared his experience on construction, I doubt that I would have shared his confidence.

The first thing the carpenter (now the foreman) wanted was a couple of professional helpers. A number of my friends worked with him, too, at greatly reduced wages, glad (I hope) of the chance to spend a summer out of doors in the woods. In these ways wages soared to $1,000 a week. But the worst news was still to come. After two weeks, around the middle of July, 1968, not even the foundations had been finished. In all, the project was to take two and a half months. Long before that time, I ran out of money.

No problem, I told myself. The bank would surely lend me what I needed.

But they wouldn't.

Their reasoning went something like this: So I was making money by teaching yoga; so, maybe a few people were crazy enough to study this absurd "science," but after all, one can't fool all the people all of the time; the yoga fad was bound to pass, and, if one was to have any faith in human nature at all, one surely couldn't expect such madness to last out the year.

For me, their rejection was a major blow. We had a temple, a common dome (kitchen, dining room, and living room), bathhouse, office, and my home all under construction, and it was imperative that they be finished before the winter storms ruined them. But the next thing I knew, the foreman and one of his two professional helpers had walked off the job. The third carpenter remained loyal, but we still had bills outstanding that amounted to thousands of dollars. Only to complete the construction was to cost me at least another $12,000. I was just screwing up my courage to try to raise this amount when the local lumber company placed a lien on the land. (So now I learned what a lien was! Years of life in a monastery had not prepared me for certain things.)

I persuaded my various creditors to accept partial monthly payments. My past record of prompt payment was an advantage. Even so, however, the least that I was able to get them to accept totaled $2,500 a month, for five months. In addition to this sum I had all my other normal expenses: apartment, car, books and correspondence office, classes, food, etc. My years in a monastery, with an allowance of $20 a month, had not prepared me for this, either!

Or had they? Knowledgeable effort alone could not possibly have taken me over this hurdle. The only thing that seems to work in times of real crisis is faith in God. I plunged in, doing the best I could, and placed the outcome wholly in His hands.

More students than ever enrolled in my classes. Friends helped generously, even nobly. Every month, several times with very little to spare, my commitments of $2,500 were paid, and all my other expenses met. At one point the lumber company, which I had been paying regularly according to our agreement, tried anyway to force a foreclosure. Miraculously, a day or two later a complete stranger came up to me after a slide show I had presented to a small group at a private home.

"I like what you're doing," he remarked. "I have a few of the world's goods. If you'll allow me to, I'd like to share a little of them with you."

"I'd be grateful for anything you gave," I said, expecting a donation of five or ten dollars. He handed me a check for $3,000!

I phoned the lumber company the next morning. "I have the money," I said, "to pay off my entire debt to you. But since you have broken our agreement, I'll let you incur all the legal fees you can, then pay you at the last moment."

"Say!" cried the owner. "If you'll agree to pay right away, I'll give you a big discount."

After paying off that debt and meeting my other expenses, I was left at the end of the month with $1.37 in my bank account!

By the end of the year, the retreat had been not only built, but very nearly paid off. People were beginning to "rally round." It was time to begin thinking seriously once again about forming our community.

43

Ananda's Founding

AS EARLY AS the end of 1967 a friend had volunteered to stay at Ananda and act as caretaker. By late summer, 1968, we were holding our first retreats in the barely completed buildings. Through the winter of that year several persons were already living at the retreat as hermits.

It was February, 1969, that we held our second meeting in San Francisco to discuss forming a community. By this time, interest and confidence in the venture had grown strong. The question was no longer whether, but *how*, to begin. The decisions reached in that second meeting, and in others that followed shortly after it, were the real beginning of Ananda Village. By the spring of 1969 the first families began arriving at Ananda. I moved there myself at the end of June. By the time I got there, it was apparent already that we would need more land.

It was in that same month that we contracted to buy a 280-acre farm six miles up the road from the retreat. Here we would develop the main part of our community, reserving the retreat primarily for classes, spiritual services, and group meditations.

The late nineteen-sixties must have been an astral hour for the founding of communities. Thousands were started during those years. All but a handful failed, most of them very quickly. I knew little or nothing about this burgeoning movement, but a movement it was, and soon the news began to spread by an amazingly efficient underground grapevine that a new "commune" had been started, and that it needed members. One afternoon alone, seven cars were lined up in our farm driveway, each of them full of people wanting to join Ananda. Many of this horde were the usual drop-outs—seekers, not for a positive way of life, but for a soft berth. They ate our food, ran up our phone bill, and told us in superior tones how we ought to be living. Most of them required at least some of our time and attention. A few of them, of course, we actually wanted as members.

For of course we did need members. What we didn't need was an invasion. We had to get the word out as quickly as possible by the ever-efficient grapevine that Ananda was not at all "where it's at." It took a while, but we were relieved at last to find ourselves being dubbed in certain circles as "up tight," materialistic (because we gave thought to paying our bills), not a real "commune." In short, Ananda began to develop its own "image"; increasingly, those who came even as visitors were to be those who were in tune with us.

The first years were certainly the hardest. People had the most unrealistic expectations. With a mortgage of $2,000 a month, they seemed to think our bills would be paid by money descending like manna from heaven, while they spent their days bucolically, dancing or lying in flowery meadows, or swimming in the nearby Yuba River, or, occasionally making a graceful gesture or two (our head gardener's description of their attempts at work) among the vegetables in the garden. When I urged them to develop businesses that would help us to meet our expenses, they looked at me indignantly as though I were prompting them to become rank materialists. If I wanted to go out and give classes to pay off the land, well, that was my "thing"; not everyone could be spiritual. But it was certainly wrong of me to ask them to join me in such sordid activities.

Was swimming in the river, I wondered, more spiritual than caring responsibly for the blessings God had given us? One of the hardest tests I had to face during that period of my life was the necessity for earning so much money, simply to make Ananda possible. But the reward, eventually, for having done so was spiritual, far more than material. I learned, then, that when we act to please God, not self, everything we do becomes a vehicle for the divine flow. For nothing, in the last analysis, is material; everything is God. Moreover, when we put out the energy necessary to overcome whatever obstacles face us in our path, we ourselves gain in strength and energy. As Master put it, a boxer doesn't grow stronger by boxing weaklings.

But many of our members of those days, typically of the youth culture then, smiled vaguely at every practical suggestion, gazed into the distance, and said, "All is God," using this divine truth to excuse the wooliest possible conclusions. Since all is God, they meant to say, He will take care of us no matter what we do—or don't do. Since all is God, our least desire must be His will, and anything we want must necessarily, therefore, be right and good. In those days, I had only to make a suggestion for half the community virtually to rise up in arms against me.

Thank God for the responsible members that came to us! I concentrated on working with them, rather than waste precious years on the play-devotees.

One of the delusions of that era, as indeed of our century, was the belief that a perfect outer setting will produce inner perfection. Thus, most "new-age" communities (as they came to be called) concentrated on outward reforms, whether in the sense of total non-possession of personal property, or of calling the land God's and opening it up to anyone who wanted to live on it, or of developing alternate sources of energy. Since I myself was convinced (and in fact the yoga teachings insist) that people must work to develop their own perfection, I had little interest in these outward "gimmicks." "Nature," according to an axiom of biology, "never makes sudden leaps." Certainly this is true of human nature. My concern was to offer people the encouragement of a way of life in which they could most easily work to perfect themselves spiritually.

I developed, therefore, a way of life that was not radically different from that which people had lived before coming to Ananda, with the added dimension of spiritual orientation. I encouraged free enterprise, private ownership of personal belongings, and individual savings. People worked for wages, and paid from their wages a certain amount to the community each month for mortgage and maintenance. They built their own homes, and continued, as they had in "the world," to cherish their own privacy. Thus, Ananda evolved as a spiritual village, rather than as a commune. People who came to us were able to adjust to this way of life more or less easily, and to focus their creative energies more fully on their own inward, spiritual development.

Critics of Ananda pointed to the higher "idealism" of other communities that made drastic demands of their members. To such critics, it seemed that we had sold out to "bourgeois America." But after all, so-called "bourgeois" America has managed, somehow, to produce the most dynamic society in the world. I don't think our success as a nation is due only to our natural resources. I think it is due primarily to our system of free enterprise. I don't see those countries which emphasize strong central planning and supervision anywhere near as successful. Nor do I see any movement in history to have succeeded remarkably that did not emphasize the principle of individual responsibility. Those communities which our critics praised have long since, and almost without exception, failed. But Ananda has grown to be widely recognized as perhaps the most successful "new-age" community in the world. Nor is its fame rooted in its material success. There are other communities that have more land, still others more money, and others, again, more members; in each case not much or not many more, for the notable successes in this movement are still only a handful. But what people speak about when referring to Ananda is the spirit of its members: their joy, their openness to others, their willingness to serve God first in everything. By giving them a way of life that they could relate to and understand, it has been possible to inspire them to grow naturally, and far beyond what they would have achieved had their spiritual growth been forced artificially, by outward means. Inevitably, I think, more and more new communities are accepting this more common-sense way of development.

But there were days, during Ananda's beginnings, when I was sorely tempted to seek once again that seclusion I had wanted for myself.

Indeed, Ananda's growth was to a large extent conditioned by this desire. I was not the kind of leader who enjoyed being constantly in the thick of things, helping Mary to overcome her annoyance with John, or Dick to work out his problems with the children. Though I am technically the chairman of our village council, the last council meeting I attended was years ago. I have preferred giving people the incentive to work out their problems on their own. Decentralization has always seemed, to me, an important organizational principle. At Ananda we try to solve problems as close to their source as possible. Not only has it given me, personally, the freedom to write, and to develop inwardly, but it has developed competent leaders within the community. These leaders will, I believe, in time, be knowledgeable enough to found similar communities elsewhere.

In time, I truly believe, "world-brotherhood colonies" will spread, as Master once put it, "like wildfire." For to my mind this is the most sensible way to live, especially for those who seek a spiritual way of life.

One of the fundamental needs of our age is for putting down roots again. We have extended ourselves too far outward from the Self within, and away from the natural rhythms of the planet on which we live. Even in our outward, human associations we have lost touch with reality. It has been estimated that the average person in America moves fourteen times in his life—and not to new homes in the same community, but to different communities altogether. Loneliness has become chronic. Friendships tend to be of the cocktail party and patio barbecue variety, and not the deep bonds that people form as a result of trials and victories shared. We know people to smile at, but not to weep with, not to confide in, not to go to for help in times of physical, emotional, or spiritual stress. Small, spiritual villages offer a viable alternative to the depersonalizing influences of our times. People living and working together, sharing with one another on many levels of their lives, suffering, growing, learning, rejoicing, and winning victories together, develop a depth in their outward relationships as well that helps them, inwardly, to acquire spiritual understanding.

This is not the book to go into all the problems of founding communities. I refer interested readers to my handbook, mentioned earlier: *Cooperative Communities—How to Start Them, and Why.* That book contains also the full story of Ananda's founding. Suffice it here to describe Ananda as, in many ways, a complete village, with schools, businesses (some of them privately owned, others owned by the community), farm, dairy, monastic as well as family areas, a public retreat, and a far-flung "Circle of Joy" which consists of friends of Ananda in many parts of the world who feel themselves spiritually a part of our family.

For the message of Ananda, finally, is not, "Come here and live with us." Rather, what we want to say to people is, "The way of life that we are demonstrating in Ananda's living laboratory, and the means to that way of life, are something that *you* can incorporate into your own life, wherever you live.''

Often I have felt Master's smile in my heart to see his "world-brotherhood colony" dream a material reality. His blessings on the land, an almost tangible aura of peace, are felt by all who come here.

And my dome home is standing solidly.

44

Conclusion

AS I GAZE OUT over Ananda's green fields, woods, and rolling hills, I sometimes think of a poem I wrote in Charleston, South Carolina, not long before coming to Master. Since then I have set it in the legendary golden era of Lord Rama, whose kingdom of Ayodhya, in ancient India, was a place of universal harmony, brotherhood, and peace. Thus may all men learn how to live, wherever their paths may take them outwardly. For now, as then, true, divine peace is possible only when people place God, and spiritual values, first in their lives.

Ayodhya in June

Listen! Fair June is humming in the air,
And Ram's Ayodhya sings of lasting peace.

The growing grass nods heavy to the wind,
Patient till cutting time. The hay is stored;
The fields spring up with adolescent plants,
Laughing flowers, berries, and graceful corn.
In the orchards, every hand is quickly busy
To catch the ripest fruits before they fall.
Men's hearts are strong with that perfected strength
That smiles at fences, lays aside old hates,
Nurtures true love, and finds such earnest pleasure
In seeking truth that every private mind
Seems drawn to virtue, like a public saint.
The women's words are soft with kindliness;
The children answer with humility;
Even the men are like so many fawns,
Modest and still, sweet with complete respect.
June in Ayodhya is so roused with joy
The earth can scarcely keep its boundaries,
Swelling with energy and waking strength
Till not a mountain, not a valley sleeps,
Straining to burst, and flood the world with laughter.

Such harmony flows everywhere when men,
With grateful hearts, offer their works to God.
Then brotherhood needs no enforcing laws,
No parliaments, no treaties sealed in fear:

True peace is theirs to whom the Lord is near.

Musing on these words, I recall with gratitude the many people here whose lives exemplify its meaning so beautifully. Embodiments they seem to me, truly, of Babaji's words to Sri Yukteswar in *Autobiography of a Yogi*: "I perceive potential saints in America and Europe, waiting to be awakened."

By odd coincidence, as I write these concluding lines it is my birthday: May 19, 1976. Exactly fifty years have passed since the life here chronicled began. Community festivities celebrating the event have, in one form or another, taken up most of the day. This afternoon, gazing on the smiling faces that were gathered around me in blessing, I thought of our Divine Beloved whose love they reflected. "Blessed are they," I quoted, "who come in the name of the Lord!"

It is evening now. I sit peacefully in my home. My gaze takes in an expansive view through the large living-room window: hills, sky, and slowly wakening stars. Such, I reflect, is the Path: Wherever man stands upon it, his soul-evolution stretches out before him to infinity. The stages on the spiritual journey are only temporary. Temporary, too, are its tests, as also its fulfillments. God alone is real.

"Divine Mother," I pray silently, "may I never become attached to Thy dream of creation, nor yet to the path that leads out of the dream, but only to Thee: to Thy love, to Thy eternal joy!"

Dear Reader:

If you've enjoyed this book, perhaps you'd like to read the complete version. Almost three times as long, it contains literally hundreds more stories and sayings—delightful, inspiring, wise—of Paramhansa Yogananda. It also offers many, many additional insights into vital aspects of the spiritual path.

The complete version of *The Path* is available in two editions: hardcover, and paperback. Please check your local bookstore: if the edition you want isn't in stock, no doubt they'd be happy to order it for you. On the other hand, if you prefer, you may place your order directly with us.

Ananda Publications was created many years ago by Swami Kriyananda to help bring his dream of Ananda Cooperative Village to fulfillment. We are part of a non-profit religious corporation; as such we also welcome donations (tax exempt) for our work. Should you care to include a free-will donation with your order, we'd be happy to send you an autographed copy of your book or books.

Joy to you!

Ananda Publications
14618 Tyler Foote Road
Nevada City, CA 95959

About the Author

SWAMI KRIYANANDA is one of the best known modern exponents of the ancient science of yoga. He is a gifted lecturer, author, teacher, composer, singer and philosopher, as well as an artist, photographer, and businessman. A Westerner trained in the Eastern teachings, he brings to his writing a clear, logical mind, down-to-earth common sense, and an ability to clarify difficult truths. Educated in Rumania, Switzerland, England and the United States, he speaks nine languages, and lectures in five of them.

Since 1962 he has written many books, short stories, plays and poems. Each of these approaches the question of life's deeper meaning from a different perspective: philosophy (*Crises in Modern Thought*); sociology (*Cooperative Communities*); psychology and astrology (*Your Sun Sign as a Spiritual Guide*); art (*Meaning in the Arts*); drama and humor ("The Jewel in the Lotus"); and the classic science of yoga (*The Path*; *Yoga Postures for Self-Awareness*; and *Fourteen Steps to Perfect Joy*).

In addition to his writing, Swami Kriyananda is also well-known for the power and quality of his voice, both as a speaker and a singer. A prolific composer, he has written original spiritual music for voice, piano and chorus. One of his current directions is "spiritualizing the arts."

It was no doubt with these accomplishments in mind that *New Directions* magazine, in Vancouver, B.C., stated, "Swami Kriyananda is perhaps the most respected non-Indian yoga exponent in the world."

How-To-Live Books
from Ananda Publications*

Cooperative Communities—How to Start Them and Why

Swami Kriyananda. paper, 120 pgs., ISBN: 0-016124-01-0, $4.95

The blueprint for a new lifestyle built on self-sufficiency, dignity and simplicity. Text includes a history of communities, their social relevance in modern civilization, and guidelines for establishing a community enterprise. Also includes the story of Ananda Cooperative Village, one of the most successful intentional communities in the world.

Crises in Modern Thought

Swami Kriyananda. paper, 248 pgs. ISBN: 0-916124-13-7, $4.95

A major contribution to the field of Western philosophy, Crises in Modern Thought confronts the modern challenge of meaninglessness with several daring challenges of its own. Without bias, Kriyananda examines nihilism, the relativity of values, the dethroning of Reason, the accidental nature of evolution, and the question of progress in evolution.

The Road Ahead

S. Kriyananda. paper, 144 pgs., ISBN: 0-916124-23-1, $4.95

Based on Paramhansa Yogananda's predictions of coming cataclysms. Analyzes society's current collision course. Offers positive ways to prepare, both inwardly and outwardly. (Available Fall, 1981)

Meaning in the Arts

S. Kriyananda. paper, ISBN: 0-916124-13-4, $3.95

Kriyananda gives guidelines for artists, educators, students: • Art as a language • Principles for testing a work of art • Analysis of music: melody, harmony, rhythm; religious music East and West • Elements of genius.

"I am now using the book as a basic text in all my classes, as well as in my own studio."—Joan Brown, MFA, Professor of Art, University of California at Berkeley. (Available Fall, 1981)

*Available at book stores or order directly from Ananda Publications. Please use order form at the back of this book.

The Art of Creative Leadership

Swami Kriyananda. paper, 16 pgs., ISBN: 0-0916124-20-7, $2.00

A helpful booklet of rules based on the premise, "People are more important than things." Presents the basic concept of how to work with people to inspire rather than drive. Especially useful for those in management positions, and useful for all who aspire to lead.

How to Spiritualize Your Marriage

S. Kriyananda. paper, 96 pgs. ISBN: 0-916124-22-3, $3.95

"They married, and lived happily ever after." How often have couples faced marriage with this romantic expectation. And how often, judging from the modern statistics on divorce, have their dreams been disappointed.

This book talks about the spiritual aspects of marriage: the right expectations, the right kinds of behavior, and marriage as something more than an end in itself. If you build marriage sensitively and truly, it will carry you past the portals of this life into eternity. Here are the principles for growing spiritually through any close relationship—for married and unmarried alike.

Your Sun Sign as a Spiritual Guide

Swami Kriyananda. paper, 129 pgs., ISBN: 0-916124-02-9, $4.95

The use of astrology as originally intended—as a science for self-discovery. Analysis of each sign is presented in terms of developing one's highest potential. Opens up the spiritual dimension of astrological counseling.

Yoga Postures for Self Awareness

Swami Kriyananda. paper, 102 pgs., many photos, ISBN: 0-916124-00-2, $4.95

A yoga primer that adds a whole new dimension to yoga practice. Its unique "awareness" approach teaches how to use body, mind, emotions, and spiritual nature for a more enjoyable life. Full-page photographs and clear instructions make this book perfect for beginners and also yoga teachers.

Stories of Mukunda

Swami Kriyananda. paper, 110 pgs., illustrated, ISBN: 0-916124-09-6, $4.95

Inspiring stories from the boyhood of Paramhansa Yogananda, yoga master and author of the classic *Autobiography of a Yogi.* Suitable for children and adults.

A Visit to Saints of India

Swami Kriyananda. paper, 100 pgs. ISBN: 0-916124-06-1, $3.95

A pilgrimage through spiritual India with an experienced and insightful guide. Includes portraits of Sai Baba, Anandamayee Ma, Muktananda and others.

Keys to the Bhagavad Gita

Swami Kriyananda. paper, ISBN: 0-916124-15-0, $3.95

"One can easily make this stimulating book a prelude to reading and understanding the *Bhagavad Gita*, for it makes you more aware and receptive to the strength and the all-compassing wisdom contained in the *Gita*." (Piya G. Uttam, *East and West Series*, Gita Publishing House, India) This book, based on the commentaries of Paramhansa Yogananda, unlocks the hidden, symbolic code of this ancient scripture. (Available Fall, 1981)

How to Use Money for Your Own Highest Good

S. Kriyananda. paper, 48 pgs., ISBN: 0-916124-22-3, $2.95

Here are the keys to a perfectly balanced attitude toward money. You'll learn how to develop prosperity consciousness, how to maintain prosperity through using money in the right way, how to gain and spend money rightly in order to grow spiritually.

Sharing Nature with Children

Awareness Guidebook by Joseph Bharat Cornell. paper, 143 pgs.
ISBN: 0-916124-14-2, illus. $4.95

A nature guide for teachers, parents, and counselors, recommended and used by Boy Scouts of America, National Audubon Society, National Science Teacher's Association, Girl Scouts of America.

Presents 42 games and activities designed to lead children into actual experiences with nature. Based on the principles that nature education should be simple, should involve direct experiences, and should teach values as well as facts.

The Divine Romance

An original sonata in three movements for piano, by Swami Kriyananda. 11 pp.,
$2.50

Melodic beauty and a mood of spiritual inspiration combine to make "The Divine Romance" a unique and moving musical experience. Both amateur and professional pianists will find this outstanding piano composition a joy to play.

Records and Tapes
from Ananda Recordings

Instruction in meditation, yoga postures, techniques for daily living, improving relationships, as well as a wide selection of music.

SPECIAL INTRODUCTORY TAPE
for readers of *The Shortened Path*

"How to Spiritualize Daily Life"
A collection of four short talks by Swami Kriyananda:
- How to Concentrate Your Energy for Success
- Overcoming Bad Moods
- How to Conquer an Inferiority Complex
- Flow with Life's Unavoidable Changes

14S6, 55 minutes, **$4.00**

Send for a free catalogue

Ananda Recordings
Department P
14618 Tyler Foote Road
Nevada City, CA 95959

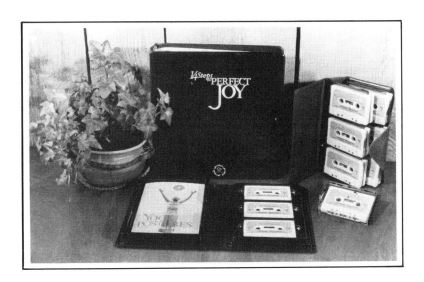

Fourteen Steps
to Perfect Joy

A Complete Program for Personal Growth
that will bring you dramatic results

Fourteen Steps to Perfect Joy is a multi-dimensional program for helping you develop your growth potential. It includes:

I. The Fourteen Steps Practice Manual

A 306-page study guide brings you hundreds of self-transforming techniques in 14 separate lessons. You receive one Step every other week for seven months, giving you two weeks to read, practice, and integrate.

II. Lessons on Tape

To enhance and reinforce your learning experience, a tape supplement accompanies each Step.

III. Personal Guidance

You can practice in the comfort of your own home and at the same time receive individual, personal guidance from specially-trained teachers and counselors.

IV. Special Course Addendum

To aid you in your practice of yoga and meditation, you receive the classic handbook on yoga, *Yoga Postures for Self-Awareness*, plus a double-cassette album of guided yoga postures plus Swami Kriyananda's new album of "Metaphysical Meditations."

You will learn how to:

- Meditate
- Heal yourself
- Develop more energy
- Eat more nutritiously and naturally
- Create a personalized schedule of yoga exercise
- Relax and relieve hypertension, fatigue and stress
- Discover and fulfill your own unique mission in life

Dramatic Results

"My job calls for a great deal of energy and patience. The techniques in the **Fourteen Steps** have not only helped in strengthening my physical will, but also they have helped me to maintain that necessary level of inner stillness while actively working in the world."

—Craig M. Dockter, Production Supervisor, Lodi, CA

Full Course $170
  (*Manual, Tapes, Addendum*)

Practice Manual Only $65

Tape Course Only $92

(*An installment payment plan is available.*)

Please write Ananda Publications for complete information.
Or call: 800-824-5993 (Outside California) • 916/265-5877 (Inside California)

Visit
Ananda Meditation Retreat

You can come to Ananda for a day, a weekend, or several months. Ananda Meditation Retreat has special-interest programs, counseling, instruction in yoga techniques and philosophy, and spiritual guidance.

The key word for retreatants is: "Relax!" Here in a peaceful forest environment you can disengage your mind from the worries and frustrations of everyday life; see and reflect on the longer rhythms of life; and look deeply to your highest Self for new energy, inspiration and solutions.

Ananda's special-interest guest programs include:

The Art of Vegetarian Cooking
Survival Awareness Workshop
Healing Seminar
Stress Without Distress/The Inner Runner
Spiritual Renewal Week

Ananda's Institute of Cooperative Spiritual Living offers longer programs (5 weeks to 3 months) including a general apprenticeship within the larger Ananda community, How-to-Live Schools Teacher Training Program, the Hermitage Program, and the Yoga Teacher Training Course.

Ananda Meditation Retreat is open to visitors every day of the year. Please write or call in advance for reservations. Send for our free detailed brochure.

Ananda Meditation Retreat
Department P
14618 Tyler Foote Road
Nevada City, CA 95959
or call:
800-824-5993 (Outside California) • 916/265-5877 (Inside California)